Weight Training for Strength and Fitness

D1501115

The Jones and Bartlett Series in Health and Physical Education

Weight Training for Strength and Fitness

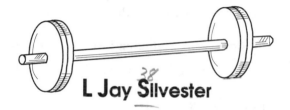

L Jay Silvester

Brigham Young University
Department of Physical Education—
Exercise Science

Jones and Bartlett Publishers
Boston   London

Editorial, Sales, and Customer Service Offices

Jones and Bartlett Publishers
One Exeter Plaza
Boston, MA 02116

Jones and Bartlett Publishers International
PO Box 1498
London W6 7RS
England

Library of Congress Cataloging-in-Publication Data
Silvester, L. Jay.
    Weight training for strength and fitness. L. Jay Silvester.
       p.   cm.
    Includes index.
    ISBN 0–86720–139–8
    1. Weight training. 2. Physical fitness. I. Title.
GV546.S55   1991
613.7'13--dc20
                                                      91-32015
                                                          CIP

Design and Production: Karen Mason
Illustrations: Lorraine Conger Cryer

Photo Credits:
Figures 1–2, Louis Cyr, and Figure 1–3, Eugene Sandow, courtesy of Todd-
    McLean Physical Culture Collection, University of Texas, Austin, Texas
Figure 1–4, Bob Hoffman and weightlifters courtesy of Mary Downie Freeman
Figure 1–5, male bodybuilder courtesy of Jay McNabney, Paradise Health Spa,
    American Fork, Utah

Printed in the United States of America
95 94 93 92   10 9 8 7 6 5 4 3 2

Contents

Chapter Three

Weight Training and Physical Fitness 41

Chapter Four

Strength Fitness and Bodybuilding (Body Sculpting) 65

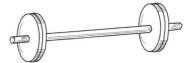

Preface

*W*eight Training for Strength and Fitness provides a reasonably detailed look at the entire spectrum of strength training. The beginner will find the material enlightening and very helpful in designing programs as well as considering which direction his or her training might go after the beginning stages have been completed. The intermediate to advanced student, teacher, or coach will enjoy the thorough coverage of the subject. Of particular interest to the reader are the concepts presented in the body building and high-level strength training sections. By reading and studying the entire text, you will have a thorough understanding of strength and strength fitness.

Chapter One is a brief presentation of the history of strength building which includes attitudes toward strength in ancient times, Olympic lifting, powerlifting, bodybuilding, strength research, and strength fitness. Significant time periods in strength history are referred to as eras, an approach that makes the subject both enjoyable and manageable.

Chapter Two contains a review of many current theories in strength training. A review of current muscle contraction theory is followed by a discussion of fiber types, motor units, summation, and synchronization. Other discussions include strength curves, strength training equipment, and speed of contraction while lifting. Overload, called here *progressive loading,* and set-repetition combinations for optimal strength and fitness are discussed. Periodization or cycling is discussed in detail using Selyes' General Adaptation Syndrome as the basis. Delayed muscle soreness, rest or recovery between sets, and exercises and ergogenic aids (particularly androgenic-anabolic steroids) are thoroughly described.

Chapter Three is devoted to weight training and physical fitness. A look at the general fitness level of Americans is followed by a suggestion to exercise by doing something enjoyable. A suggestion that being physically fit has many dimensions, including aerobic fitness, strength, muscular endurance, flexibility, and proper body composition (attention to proper nutrition), ends this chapter.

Chapter Four examines strength fitness exercise bodybuilding and body sculpting. Strength fitness exercise is the workout for the masses. Example programs are presented. Working to momentary muscular failure is discussed as is working at or close to fatigue levels. Two bodybuilders are followed through a day's routine to get an idea of the intensity of their workouts. Muscular hypertrophy and body types are examined.

Chapter Five examines the strength training of athletes, Olympic weightlifters, and powerlifters—all are considered among those engaged in high-level strength training. Specificity of training, both physiological and biomechanical, is discussed along with strength and athletic performance. The reader should not expect that increased strength will automatically result in increased ability in one's chosen sport. However, strength profiles for success in any sport can be developed; and one for an international class discus thrower is presented. Plyometric exercise is also thoroughly covered. Competitive lifting, which includes descriptions of the lifts and training programs, is presented for both the Olympic and powerlifter.

In Chapter Six, beginning and advanced periodized weight training programs (three-phase) are outlined. These represent excellent examples of workouts to follow.

Chapter Seven describes the execution of a number of strength training exercises. The primary muscles involved in each exercise are identified. A skeletal view of the muscles is presented at the end of the chapter.

Chapter Eight is useful as a gauge of personal ability. There is no claim to extreme reliability or validity. These criteria may be used to understand where one stands relative to standards developed over a period of time.

From ancient to modern times, from the once-per-week fitness advocate to the intense competitive lifter who trains three times per day, from scientific theory to "just lift and you'll get stronger," this book covers strength training in a complete and unique manner. May all who read this text learn from it as well as enjoy its benefits.

ACKNOWLEDGMENTS

No textbook is ever writen without the assistance of a number of individuals. Those who were most instrumental in bringing this work to fruition are acknowledged here:

First to my wife and sweetheart, a grateful thank you for the hours of endurance and many words and signs of encouragement.

To Lorraine Conger Cryer, whose deft hand and mind created all of the drawings in this book. A sincere thank you with attendent admiration for your talent.

To Terry and Jan Todd of the Iron Game Library at the University of Texas; Mrs. Mary Freema; Jim Wright, Associate Editor of *Muscle and Fitness* Magazine; and Ms. Sherrie Byttle, my gratitude for allowing me to use photographs which were and are essential to the proper completion of this book.

To Kartsi Lappaluotto and Brent Patera, the very excellent models for the Olympic and powerlifting photographs. My thanks for your skill and your photogenic qualities.

To Don Norton of the English Department of Brigham Young University, my thanks for proofing and improving the manuscript. The book reads much better because of you.

To Karen Mason, the design and production service, my gratitude for endurance, kindness, and a fine job well executed.

Weight Training for Strength and Fitness

CHAPTER ONE

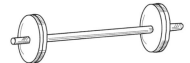

A Brief Look at the Past

We consider the past because doing so is interesting and informative to those who are intellectually curious. If you are a practitioner who wants only a workout routine and has no concern for any tangents to strength or bodybuilding, turn to Chapter Two.

What brought us to our current state of understanding and practice in weight training? Who were the central figures in strength building, and what did they profess? You will find answers to these and many other questions on the following pages. Our journey through the ages is intentionally brief but uniquely informative, even intriguing.

THE ANCIENT ERA

The origin of weight training is lost in antiquity. It is a given that great strength was necessary for survival in ancient times, and it is also safe to assume that men from our most distant past competed with one another in strength contests.

There is evidence that some form of weightlifting was practiced in ancient Egypt, Ireland, China, and Greece. Paintings on the walls of Egyptian tombs give ample evidence that the people participated in all manner of physical activities. Two pictures found in an Egyptian tomb and dated about 2500 B.C. depict strength developing exercises. The "wheel feat," a form of weight throwing, was contested in Irish games as early as 1829 B.C. In China during the latter part of the Chou Dynasty (1122–255 B.C.) a special military examination included a test to determine how much weight a prospective soldier could lift (8) .

The ancient Greeks may not have been any more interested in feats of strength than other societies of that era, but they did record more about such activity. A 315-pound red sandstone block found at Olympia carries the inscription that in the sixth century B.C. A Greek named Bybon threw the boulder over his head with one hand! A larger boulder (1058 pounds), found at Santorin and inscribed in the sixth century B.C., stated that Emastus, son of Critobulus, lifted it clear of the ground (8).

Milo of Crotona (Figure 1–1) is certainly the most famous of ancient Greek strongmen. He started developing his strength by shouldering a calf each day and carrying it a few yards across the barnyard. Milo continued lifting the animal daily until it reached maturity! His most famous strength achievement was lifting a four-year-old heifer onto his shoulders and then carrying it the length of the Stadium at Olympia, a distance of approximately 200 yards. Titormus, an Aetolian shepherd, ultimately defeated Milo in a boulder lifting contest and further displayed his prowess by holding two wild bulls fast by the heels (8). (Incidentally, the tale of

Figure 1–1
Milo strength
training

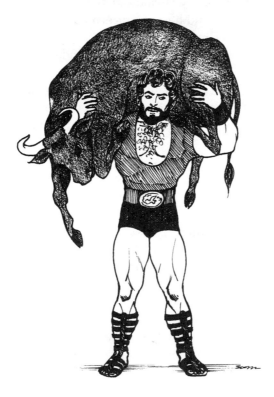

Milo's demise records that while he was walking through a forest he noticed a tree stump with a wedge imbedded in it. The idea of removing the wedge with his bare hands became a personal challenge that he could not resist. Sometime during the struggle, the wedge fell free but his hand or hands became caught in the stump. Trapped by the stump, he ultimately became a meal for wild animals.)

➤ *Would Milo's system of strength training be a useful method for athletes of the 1990s?*

The ancient Greeks also appreciated personal fitness and beauty. Young Spartan men between the ages of eighteen and twenty were periodically required to parade naked before a panel of *ephors* (state officials) who judged their fitness and appearance. Those who were not up to standard were whipped by the *ephors* and encouraged to be better the next time (13). Such consequences for lack of fitness were perhaps extreme but as far as we know they were effective. Van Dalen suggests of the ancient Athenians, "No other people were possesed of such personal beauty and no other people so much appreciated the gift" (13).

THE ERA OF PROFESSIONAL STRONGMEN AND STRENGTH QUACKERY

During the late 1800s and through the first decade of the twentieth century, professional strongmen were popular in both Europe and the United States. Such men toured through these countries with circuses or vaudeville troupes, putting on shows that were a combination of strength and chicanery.

Richard Pennel, who is credited with being the originator of the strongman movement in the America, made weightlifting history in 1870 by pushing overhead, in one hand, 201 1/4 pounds (8).

Louis Cyr (Figure 1–2), a 300-pound French Canadian, is reputed to have lifted 987 pounds clear of the floor with one hand; to have pressed 273 1/4 pounds with one hand; and, gripping a bar with only his hands (using no harness or straps), to have lifted 1897 pounds clear of the floor (8).

Perhaps the greatest showman among these early strength merchants was the famed Eugene Sandow (Figure 1–3). In one remarkable stunt he used a bar with brass spheres three feet in diameter on the ends. With great effort Sandow would raise the bar overhead with one arm and when an assistant would release a man from each bell, drop it suddenly, catch it with both hands, and lower it lightly to the floor. The total weight has been estimated at about 320 pounds (8).

Figure 1–2
Louis Cyr—in his day, one of the strongest men on earth

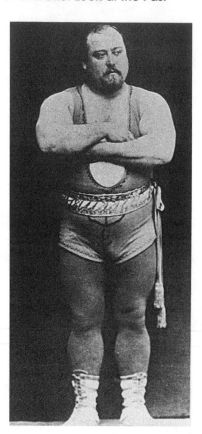

Figure 1–3
Eugene Sandow, whose physique and showmanship gave rise to bodybuilding in the United States

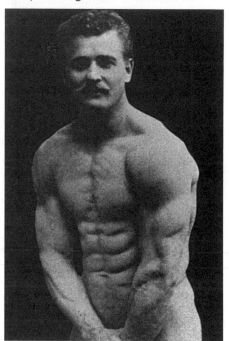

One of Sandow's most impressive and well-documented feats occurred while he was being examined by the famed Dr. Dudley Sargent. Becoming a bit bored by pulling on a dynamometer, the strongman informed those present that he would show them a real feat of strength. He then asked who was the largest man in the room; it happened to be Dr. Sargent at 175 pounds. Sandow then knelt down and placed his hand at arm's length, palm up, on the floor and asked Dr. Sargent to climb aboard with one foot. He easily lifted Dr. Sargent from the floor to a table top while keeping his arm straight (8)!

Eugene Sandow, the best known of the strength showmen, is the person whose image gave rise to bodybuilding in the United States.

Many of these early strength merchants were large, somewhat obese men whose movements were not the most fluid. People who saw them perform came to associate weightlifting with awkwardness and ponderosity. These early lifters must be credited with contributing to, if not being the major perpetrators of, the concept of muscle-boundness, a condition which could be described as a combination of awkwardness and inflexiblity. The association of weightlifting and muscle-boundness persists in the minds of some to this day even though most athletes on collegiate and professional teams use strength training as part of their conditioning.

In addition to contributing to the muscle-bound concept, early strongmen often made false claims about their strength and frequently staged shows that were characterized by trickery and deception. Such conduct ultimately caused considerable public distrust and rejection.

Strength showmen of the eighteenth and early nineteenth centuries must be credited with contributing to, if not being the major perpetrators of, the concept of muscle-boundness.

The total impact of these strongmen on our society is not clear. Certainly they entertained many people during their time with their great physical prowess, and they must be considered a link in the history of the physically strong. Just as certainly, however, they created an aversion for strength training in the minds of most Americans. From about 1910 to the late 1940s, strength training was thought to be an activity for only cultish bodybuilders trying to improve their appearance and self-image and a few curious strongmen who definitely did not inspire many others to become like them.

➤ *Does weightlifting cause an individual to become muscle-bound?*

COMPETITIVE WEIGHTLIFTING

Olympic-Style Weightlifting

Weightlifting has been contested in all the Olympic Games since 1896. The first American to win a weightlifting championship in an Olympic Game was Otto C. Osthoff, at the St. Louis Olympics in 1904. He won the dumbbell competition. In those same Olympics, Fred Winters was the first American to set a world record. His record was in the two-hand dumbbell press (7).

> Otto C. Osthoff, who won the dumbbell competition in the
> 1904 Olympic Games at St. Louis, Missouri, was the first
> American to win an Olympic weightlifting championship
> for the United States.

After that, however, no American competed in weightlifting at the Olympic Games until 1932. The cost of getting to the Games and the relative unpopularity of the sport were considerations that kept Americans out of Olympic weightlifting.

In 1928 the first United States weightlifting championships were held in the Los Angeles Coliseum. In 1929 the Amateur Athletic Union (AAU) sponsored the first senior national weightlifting championships at the German-American Athletic Club in New York City (7).

In 1932 the International Olympic Committee standardized the Olympic lifts. The three lifts used in the competition from then until 1972 were the two-hands snatch, the two-hands clean and press, and the two-hands clean and jerk. In 1972 the two-hands clean and press was eliminated as an Olympic lift because it had become essentially another jerk.

At about this same time (1932), the father of Olympic-style weightlifting in the United States, Robert (Bob) Hoffman, became a major force in U.S. and international weightlifting. More than any other person in the United States, he has contributed time, money, and heart to building up the sport he loved. In his younger years he was an active lifter who competed in a variety of strongman contests. Bob organized the York, Pennsylvania, Barbell Club in 1932. His financial success from selling weightlifting equipment and health foods enabled him to support himself and others who lifted and worked at the York complex (7).

> Bob Hoffman has contributed more time, money, and
> heart to Olympic-style weightlifting than any other person
> in the history of the United States.

Bob wanted the best athletes around him, so he recruited them from all across the United States. His method of recruiting amounted to offering good lifters a job in York, Pennsylvania, the best in training facilities, and time to train and compete. Those were rather irresistible offers to most lifters of that era. Teams representing his interests won fifty senior national weightlifting championships from 1929 through 1980 (7).

War took precedence over sport from 1939 to 1945 as the world struggled with oppression. Neither world championships nor Olympic Games were conducted during those years. In 1946 and 1947, however, the United States, because of the dedication of Bob Hoffman and those training with him, won the world title in weightlifting for the first and second times (7).

At the 1948 Olympic Games in London, the United States won their first of three team championships in Olympic weightlifting. The 1948 team won comfortably ahead of second place, but the next two Olympic championships were won by the narrowest of margins. In 1952 Americans beat the Soviet Union by only one point, and in the 1956 Olympics in Melbourne, Australia, the point total for the United States and the Soviet Union was tied but the Americans won because they had four gold medals and the Soviets had only three. All three wins occurred with Bob Hoffman as team coach–manager.

Some of the lifters whose efforts contributed to the U.S. superiority during this time period were Anthony Terlazzo (148 lbs.), John Davis (heavyweight), Tommy Kono (181 lbs.), Joseph Depietro (123 lbs.), Frank Spellman (165 lbs.), Stanley Stanczyk (181 lbs.), Norbert Schemansky (198 lbs.), Chuck Vinci (123 lbs.), Isaac Berger (132 lbs.), and the great Paul Anderson (heavyweight). The phenomenal, John Davis who won a world championship in Vienna, Austria, at age 17 (181-lb. class) won two Olympic Golds—

Figure 1-4
The York Barbell team of the 1950s. (l–r): Tommy Kono, Clyde Emrich, Stanley Stanczyk, Coach Robert Hoffman, John Davis, Norbert Schemansky, and Dave Sheppard.

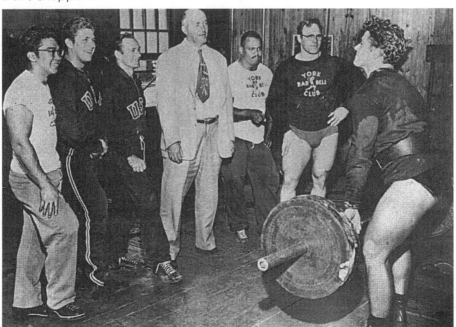

1948 and 1952—in the heavyweight class. All other lifters listed above were Olympic victors (7).

Under Bob Hoffman's leadership the United States won three consecutive Olympic weightlifting team titles: 1948, 1952, and 1956.

The Olympic weightlifting fortunes of the United States have taken a dramatic turn downward since 1956. The reason for this dearth of U.S. Olympic lifters centers primarily around the lack of rewards for participating (financial, lifestyle, etc.) and the time required to master the very demanding techniques.

Powerlifting

As a result of American success in Olympic lifting there was an upsurge in weightlifting among athletes despite the fear of becoming "muscle-bound." However, the technical difficulty of the Olympic lifts and the fact that all such lifting ends up overhead have been major obstacles to the growth of such lifting in the United States. Not only are the Olympic lifts very demanding technically, they are generally considered quite dangerous to backs and shoulders. These factors have combined to cause athletes and others to use different lifts to develop their strength.

Athletes are very competitive, and it certainly doesn't challenge the imagination to visualize the training contests that have taken place in weight rooms around the country. At some point in time a group of lifters from one gym or school challenged another. What to call this contest? The lifts to be contested were not the Olympic lifts—they were "odd." So, the name became odd lift contest. Odd lift contests were the basis for determining just which lifts, other than the Olympic three, were best suited for competition. The three lifts (note that there were three, following the Olympic format) decided on were the parallel squat, the bench press, and the deadlift. The sport was named powerlifting, and the first national contest was conducted in 1964.

Powerlifting began as strictly an American sport, and it has since become much more popular in the United States than the Olympic-style lifting. Athletes in all sections of the United States use the powerlifts in their training. The clean has also become a very popular conditioning lift for athletes. The overhead jerk and press have not found favor with most who seek strength and power for improved sport performance.

> The United States has dominated powerlifting worldwide since its inception. No other country has seriously challenged U.S. superiority from 1964 to 1990.

The first world championships in powerlifting were held in 1971. The United States won that championship and has won all those subsequent to it through 1988. Competitors from Japan, Great Britain, Finland, and Sweden have done some exceptional lifting, but teams from those countries have not seriously threatened American dominance.

Some names of successful lifters are Dr. Terry Todd (SHW), Larry Pacifico (198 lbs.), George Frenn (242 lbs.), Jon Cole (242 lbs.), Vince Anello (198 lbs.), Ricky Dale Crain (148 lbs.), Bill Kazmier (SHW), Lamar Gant (132 lbs.), Mike Bridges (148–181 lbs.), Rick Gaughler (165 lbs.); and Dr. Fred Hatfield (220–242 lbs.).

Joe Zarella, who was elected National Powerlifting Chariman in 1977, promoted powerlifting programs for women. As a result of his and other individuals' pioneering efforts, women now participate in a number of contests throughout the world. The first U.S. national powerlifting championships for women were staged in 1978, and the first world championships took place in May, 1980.

Jan Todd, wife of Dr. Terry Todd, set many world records in powerlifting and became an articulate representative for women in strength sports when she appeared on a number of TV talk shows and later became a commentator for televised powerlifting contests. Other outstanding female powerlifters include Pam Miester (105 lbs.), United States; Bev Francis (165 lbs.), Australia; Ann Turbyne (HW), United States; and Karen Gadja (132 lbs.), United States. Any list of successful lifters is necessarily incomplete. Those mentioned are some of the greats of the beginning years.

THE BODYBUILDING ERA

Most of the weight trainers in the United States lift weights because they want to tone up or, to use the terms currently in vogue, to "buff up." These terms suggest that most people want to be muscularly fit and at the same time feel good and look good. Bodybuilders are concerned first and foremost with appearance, but they also presume, quite correctly, that their workout routines will result in very high levels of muscular fitness. Most people, in fact, are quite concerned with their appearance, perhaps more so than with strength or fitness. Not that all people want to put in the time and effort required to become an elite-class bodybuilder, but most of us would like a nice physique.

Bodybuilding, as we know it today in the United States, arose out of the professional strongman era. Eugene Sandow was the major catalyst that interested Americans in muscular, well-proportioned bodies (10). He combined great showmanship with an unusually well-developed body and surprising strength. With his first appearance in a vaudeville show promoted by Florence Ziegfeld during the 1890s, he became an overnight sensation. His feats of strength and body proportions inspired many Americans to begin lifting weights to improve their bodies.

The object of bodybuilding for men is threefold: (1) to cause muscle to hypertrophy as much as possible, (2) to balance the muscular development of the body into a symmetrical whole, and (3) to produce as much vascularity as possible.

The object of bodybuilding for women is to develop impressive muscularity but not to the degree of the men (Figure 1–5). Balance and symmetry count very much, as do poise and feminine presentation. Bodybuilders often refer to what they do as living art; thus "sculpting the body" is a common phrase in bodybuilding, particularly among women.

Figure 1–5
Male and female bodybuilders of the 1990s

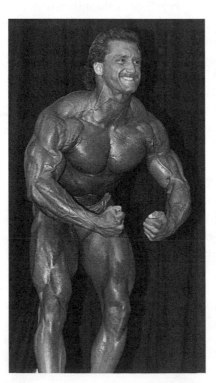
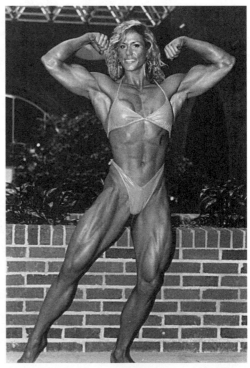

The first physique contest in the United States was held in Madison Square Garden in 1903. This contest, promoted by a businessman–promoter, Bernarr McFadden, was the only one of its type for more than twenty years. In the late 1930s the Amateur Athletic Union (AAU) assumed control of bodybuilding and put on the first Mr. America contest. Today there are many contests. The primary organizations that sponsor contests are the International Federation of Bodybuilding (IFBB), mentioned first because a competition it sponsors, Mr. Olympia, is the most prestigious in all of bodybuilding; the AAU; the World Bodybuilding Guild (WBBG); and in England, the National Amateur British Bodybuilding Association (NABBA) (10).

Some of the great bodybuilders from 1940 to the present have been Charles Atlas, John Grimek, Steve Reeves, Bill Pearl, Dave Draper, Lou Ferrigno, Franco Columbu, and perhaps the greatest, Arnold Schwarzenegger, who gave up bodybuilding for a successful career in movie making (10).

THE INFLUENCE OF DR. THOMAS DeLORME

The influence of Dr. Thomas DeLorme in bringing strength training to a state of public respectability and curiosity probably cannot be overstated. During the 1940s this physician at Massachusetts General Hospital compared recovery rates of postoperative and other impaired patients who used weight training to recovery rates of those who did not. Dr. DeLorme was himself a weightlifter and weight trainer who had begun weight training as a teenager. When he began work in rehabilitation at Massachusetts General Hospital he naturally wanted to see the results of weight training on his patients (11). The results were quite positive, and this started the process of using weight training as an effective fitness-producing modality.

> The impact of Dr. Thomas DeLorme in bringing strength training to a state of public respectability and curiosity probably cannot be overstated.

DeLorme devised the following system of weight training. First establish a ten-repetition maximum (10 RM) in your choice of exercises. Let's assume that your 10 RM in the bench press was 100 pounds. The workout thereafter would include three sets for each exercise. The first set would consist of ten repetitions (reps) at a weight of one-half of the 10 RM (50 lbs.), the second set would be ten reps at 3/4 of the 10 RM (75 lbs.), and the last set would be ten reps at the 10 RM weight (100 lbs.) (5, 6). Although bodybuilders do not use this system it certainly was and is an effective strength fitness routine.

Because of his eminence as a medical doctor and his commitment to helping people, Dr. DeLorme was able to begin to open the American mind to the possibilities of weight training. His work encouraged others to carefully and fairly evaluate the effects of weight training on fitness and athletic conditioning. That evaluation process has led to the irrefutable conclusion that weight training is a very effective means of producing strength and other positive fitness benefits.

THE ERA OF STRENGTH RESEARCH

Subsequent to Dr. DeLorme's signal efforts in weight training, various other researchers began the process of carefully and thoroughly qualifying the effects of different weight-training techniques. Edward Capen (2), Edward Chui (3), Peter Karpovich (14), and others were instrumental in producing research results that stand as the basis for much of the current weight training theory. However, one researcher has done more than any other to develop understanding of the results of various set-repetition combinations. Dr. Richard Berger of Temple University concluded after many research studies that doing three sets of the six RM was slightly better than doing sets of eight or ten or sets of two to four RMs (1).

L. Matveyev of the Soviet Union must have been intrigued with mixing various training systems to produce a particular effect. His pioneer work in what has been dubbed periodization or cycling has resulted in a rather complex workout routine that has produced strength results slightly superior to more traditional set systems (9). John Garhammer and Dr. Michael Stone have completed research studies that show some advantage in using the periodization concept when seeking strength gains through weight training (12). As in any field of endeavor, research is an ongoing process. Undoubtedly other interesting and useful concepts will be produced by those who pursue new knowledge. However, to those of us who understand raw strength and power, the specter of Milo lifting that bull in the sixth century B.C. looms hauntingly in our minds. It may be that the system Milo used to produce strength and power cannot be improved on.

It may well be that the system Milo used to produce total body strength and power cannot be improved on.

THE ERA OF THE ATHLETE AND STRENGTH

Athletes have always recognized the value of great strength. They have also recognized the value of being supple, agile, and fast. From the 1920s through the 1950s gaining strength by weightlifting was generally thought to produce a muscle-bound person who could not move fluidly. During the first half of the twentieth century most athletes and coaches stayed away from strength training. Even after certain athletes started showing significant positive results from strength training programs no one rushed to jump on the strength training bandwagon. The fear of becoming muscle-bound held a strong grip on the American mind.

The first American athletes to wholly embrace weightlifting as a conditioning modality were the track and field throwers of the 1950s and early 1960s. While others were wondering what the effects of a strength training program might be, these men were becoming very strong. Four hundred pound bench presses, 500 to 600 pound squats, and 350 to 400 pound cleans were not uncommon among these athletes. They were engaged in an unreserved drive to become as strong as possible, which they unquestionably believed would allow them to throw greater distances than ever before. Of all the athletes who might benefit from exceptional strength (physical power), shot putters, discus throwers, and hammer throwers would probably benefit the most. Not far behind these throwers as athletes who stand to benefit from great strength, and perhaps not behind at all, are football linemen.

> The first American athletes to wholly embrace weightlifting as a conditioning modality were the track and field throwers of the 1950s and early '60s.

However, football players and coaches did not begin realizing the benefits of weight training until the early to mid 1960s. By the mid to late 1970s strength training was a mainstay in any successful university football program.

Boyd Epley, the strength and conditioning coach for the University of Nebraska, and others inaugurated the National Strength Coaches' Association (NSCA) in 1977. The name was later changed to the National Strength Conditioning Association. Today, strength training facilities are constructed for entire university athletic programs, but football programs, because of the money, popularity, and the numbers of people associated with the game, have the greatest influence on strength training at the collegiate level. Most high schools have also invested heavily in weight training facilities. Very few are without weight training setups. High school facilities are normally used by both the athletic teams and the general student population.

THE FITNESS PHENOMENON OF THE 1960s AND 1970s

It would be improper to refer to the fitness upsurge of the mid-twentieth century as an "era of fitness." Physical fitness has been considered important throughout the history of man. But there was a reawakening in the American consciousness of the benefits of exercise during the mid-twentieth century. Dr. Kenneth Cooper (4) was certainly the preeminent figure in this phenomenon. He emphasized aerobic or endurance training, but his influence stimulated all fitness activities.

Today we have weightlifters, powerlifters, bodybuilders, athletes, and rehabilitating patients lifting weights for a variety of reasons, but by far the largest group of those who lift weights in the United States are those who do it to improve their appearance, fitness, or both. This group is referred to as weight trainers. Those who want to tone up, or reduce the flabbiness of the muscle, and those who want to "buff up," meaning to put a little muscle in the right places (most people want to do both) make up most of the army of people who exercise with weights in our 1990s society.

To get an idea of the popularity of weight training in our country, first consider the number of commercial fitness establishments in the United States, then think of all the weight training classes that are taught in our schools from junior high through college, consider the apartment complexes and hotels and motels that have weight training facilities, consider how many businesses have set up conditioning facilities for their employees, and finally think about the millions of individuals who have purchased weight training equipment for themselves and their families. Not everyone lifts weights in the late-twentieth century United States, but many people do!

➤ *What are some indications of the popularity of weight training in our society?*

The United States of the 1990s is a society that is becoming increasingly sophisticated, computerized, and mechanized. A society burdened with many difficult problems—environmental pollution, drugs, unchecked federal debt, and the health and health care of our nation. Exercise, including exercise against resistance (weight training), will play an increasingly important role as our nation seeks ways to improve the health of our citizenry and contain soaring health-care costs.

REFERENCES

1. Berger, R. A. 1963. Comparative effects of three weight training programs. *Research Quarterly* 34: 396-398.
2. Capen, E. K. 1950. The effect of systematic weight training on power, strength, and endurance. *Research Quarterly* 21: 83–93
3. Chui, E. F. 1950. The effect of systematic weight training on athletic power. *Research Quarterly* 21: 188–194.
4. Cooper, K. H. 1968. *Aerobics.* New York: M. Evans Co.
5. DeLorme, T. L. 1945. Restoration of muscle power by heavy resistance exercise. *Journal of Bone and Joint Surgery* 27: 645-667.
6. DeLorme, T. L., and A. L. Watkins. 1948. Techniques of progressive resistance exericise. *Archives of Physical Medicine* 29: 263.
7. Kutzer, W. F. 1979. The history of olympic weightlifting in the United States. Doctoral dissertation. Brigham Young University.
8. Massey, B. H., H. W. Freeman, et al. 1959. *The Kinesiology of Weightlifting.* Dubuque, Iowa: Wm. C. Brown.
9. Matveyev L. 1981. *Fundamentals of Sport Training* 2nd ed. (Trans. Albert P. Zdornykh). Moscow, USSR: Progress Publishers.
10. Gaines, C., and G. Butler. 1980. *Pumping Iron; The Art and Sport of Bodybuilding* New York. Simon & Schuster.
11. Rasch, P. J. 1982. *Weight Training* 4th ed. Dubuque, Iowa: Wm. C. Brown.
12. Stone, M. H., H. O'Bryant, J. Garhammer, et al. 1982. A theoretical model of strength training. *National Strength and Conditioning Journal* 4 (4): 36–39.
13. Van Dalen, D. B., and B. L. Bennett. 1971. *A World History of Physical Education* 2nd ed. Englewood Cliffs, N. J.: Prentice-Hall.
14. Zorbas, W. S., and P. V. Karpovich. 1951. The effect of weightlifting upon the speed of muscular contractions. *Research Quarterly* 22: 145–148.

CHAPTER TWO

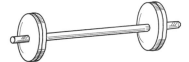

Modern Strength Training Theory

*M*odern strength training theory includes all the knowledge about strength development that is currently accepted by those who have done research in the field and have painstakingly drawn conclusions from that research. Most of these truths are discussed in this section. Some of the concepts discussed have not been confirmed through scientific research projects, but, in my opinion, merit attention.

> Modern strength training theory includes all strength training theory substantiated by research and some as-yet untested concepts.

MUSCLE ANATOMY

A skeletal muscle is made up of thousands of single muscle cells, or muscle fibers, covered with a thin cell membrane known as the *sarcolemma*. Most of these muscle fibers run the entire length of the skeletal muscle and have only one neuromuscular junction located near the midpoint (13). A single *motor neuron,* or nerve fiber, and all the muscle fibers it innervates are known as a *motor unit.* Within the intracellular fluid or *sarcoplasm,* which bathes the components of the muscle fiber, are various microscopic organelles. Two of the most notable are the contractile protein strands known as *myofibrils* and the series of tubules called the *sarcoplasmic reticulum,* which functions as a transportation and, communication system within the muscle cell. Each muscle contains several hundred to several thousand myofibrils, which are composed of the smaller protein myofilaments *actin* and *myosin* (13). Actin and myosin filaments are the basic moving *structures* in microscopic muscle contraction.

Connective tissue binds together and covers all skeletal muscle. The *endomysium* covers each muscle fiber and binds adjacent fibers. The *perimysium* surrounds and binds groups of fibers together to form a *fasciculus* or *muscle bundle.* The *epimysium* binds muscle bundles to form a whole muscle such as the triceps or pectoralis major (13, 26).

It is important to understand that connective tissue is interspersed *throughout* the muscle belly, ultimately meshing together at the ends of each muscle to form tendons. Force produced by muscle contraction is transmitted through this network of connective tissue to the tendons that are attached to the lever system of bones. Body parts move when muscular force is great enough to move the body part and overcome any associated resistance. (See Figure 2–1A.)

Microscopic Muscle Structure and Function

The basic *contractile unit* of the muscle, the sarcomere, is found in the threadlike myofibril strands. (See Figure 2–1B.) The limits of a sacromere are the filamentous proteins known as Z discs. (See Figures 2–1B and 2–1C). Between the Z discs, actin (light) and myosin (darker) myofilaments produce light and dark banding or striation. The H zone is the area between the ends of the actin filaments. In normally functioning muscle, the actin filaments within the sarcomere are seldom stretched to the extent necessary to produce an H zone (13). The I band (I is short for *isotropic,* meaning that light can pass through, however slightly) is the area occupied by actin filaments and includes the Z discs. The A band (A stands for *anisotropic,* which refers to the property of preventing light from shining through) includes both sets of myosin filaments.

Actin filaments, which are double the number of myosin filaments, are made up of two *F actin strands* wound together in a double helix. (See Figure 2–1D.) A chain of long, thin protein molecules called *tropomyosin* is bound to each F actin strand. Periodically attached to tropomyosin are molecules of an inhibitory protein known as *troponin* (13). Myosin filaments, which account for 68 percent of the protein within the sarcomere,

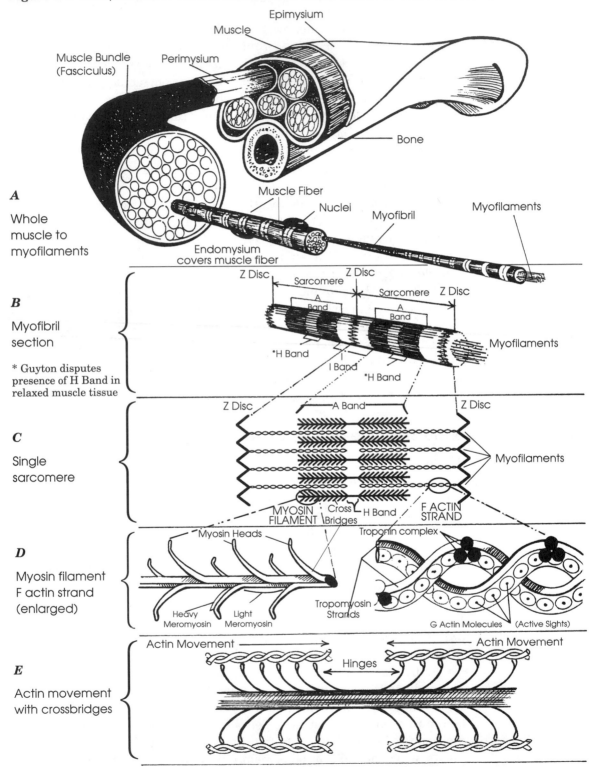

Figure 2–1 Components of skeletal muscle, from whole muscle to actin and myosin

Epimysium

Muscle

Perimysium

Muscle Bundle
(Fasciculus)

Bone

A

Whole
muscle to
myofilaments

Muscle Fiber

Nuclei

Myofibril

Myofilaments

Endomysium
covers muscle fiber

Z Disc

Z Disc

Sarcomere

Sarcomere

Z Disc

B

Myofibril
section

* Guyton disputes
presence of H Band in
relaxed muscle tissue

A
Band

A
Band

Myofilaments

*H Band

I Band

*H Band

C

Single
sarcomere

Z Disc

A Band

Z Disc

Myofilaments

MYOSIN
FILAMENT

Cross
Bridges

H Band

F ACTIN
STRAND

D

Myosin filament
F actin strand
(enlarged)

Myosin Heads

Troponin complex

Heavy
Meromyosin

Light
Meromyosin

Tropomyosin
Strands

G Actin Molecules

(Active Sights)

E

Actin movement
with crossbridges

Actin Movement

Actin Movement

Hinges

are composed of peptide molecule strands wound together to form a double helix. Myosin is further distinguished by densely woven helixes, or *heavy meromyosin*, and less dense helixes, known as *light meromyosin*. The heavy meromyosin protrudes from the myosin strands to form *cross bridges,* which are positioned in precise relationship to the surrounding actin filaments. (See Figure 2–1E.) On each cross bridge there is a globular protein mass known as the *myosin head*. The hinged movement of these myosin heads as they repeatedly contact, pull, and then release, flow back, and contact another active site on the actin strands is thought to be the mechanical process of muscle contraction this is also known as the sliding filament or rachet theory of muscle contraction (13).

BRIEF CHEMISTRY OF MUSCLE CONTRACTION

When an impulse from a motor nerve reaches a muscle fiber, the fiber membrane allows positively charged sodium ions to rush in, reversing the charge these fibers had in their resting state. This change in charge (depolarization) moves across the muscle membrane and, via the transverse tubules, deep into fiber. When the depolarization reaches special calcium storage sacs within the sarcoplasmic reticulum, calcium ions that inactivate the inhibitory protein troponin are released. When calcium levels become high enough, troponin is inactivated and myosin proteins enzymatically split adenosine triphosphate (ATP) into adensine diphosphate (ADP) and energy. This ATP-splitting activity appears to take place at the cross bridges. The energy released from ATP allows actin and myosin to cross link, and the myosin heads to return to a "cocked" position after the power stroke. (See Figure 2–1E.) However, the power stroke of the myosin heads is thought to occur independently of the energy supplied by ATP (13). When nervous stimulation stops, the calcium ions are pumped via a special chemical pump back into the sacs in the sarcoplasmic reticulum, troponin inhibits myosin activity, and the muscle relaxes (13).

MUSCLE/FIBER TYPES

Researchers have developed a technique for removing a minute plug of skeletal muscle with a special needle inserted into a muscle through a small incision in the skin. This *muscle biopsy* procedure has been used for a number of years to facilitate scientific examination of muscle tissue.

After a tissue sample has been sliced into tiny, thin pieces and stained with the proper enzymes to bring out particular colors, fibers in the sample

Table 2–1 Muscle/Fiber Types

Common muscle fiber identifying terms

Slow	Intermediate	Fast
Type I	Type IIa	Type IIb
Slow oxidative (SO)	Fast oxidative glycolytic (FOG)	Fast glycolytic (FG)
Slow twitch (ST)	Fast twitch (FT)	Fast twitch (FT)

Color

Deep red	Red	White

can be typed and counted with the use of powerful microscopes. Years of evaluation and study have resulted in agreement that there are essentially three types of skeletal muscle fibers. Muscle fibers are identified by what they look like or how they function. Perhaps the easiest way of identifying different fiber types is to refer to them as either (1) slow (2) intermediate or (3) fast. Other commonly used names for these fibers are listed in Table 2–1.

The muscles of weightlifters, throwers, sprinters, and other power event athletes often contain a high percentage of fast fibers. Conversely, the muscles of long-distance runners, skiers, cyclists, and swimmers are normally a larger percentage of slow fibers.

The fiber types that we have are generally determined by our heredity. The concept that "sprinters are born, not made" is generally true. Intense training can improve a person's ability for strength or endurance, but if the genetic capacity is not there it is very unlikely that a person could become either a extremely competent endurance athlete or a world class strength-power performer.

MOTOR UNITS, SUMMATION, SYNCHRONIZATION, AND STRENGTH

Motor units include a motor nerve and all of the muscle fibers innervated by that nerve. All the muscle fibers in a particular motor unit are of the same type. Therefore we can refer to motor units as: fast glycolytic (FG), fast oxidative glycolytic (FOG), and slow oxidative (SO). These are distinguished by the speed of their contractions and their ability to resist fatigue. The human body uses FG muscle fibers (motor units) for explosive movements such as sprinting or lifting heavy weights. We use SO fibers for standing or slow walking. FOG fibers are thought to be activated in relatively high intensity activities of longer duration than a brief weightlifting movement or sprint, such as running 300 to 500 meters (26).

When a nervous stimulus reaches what is known as *threshold* level, the muscle fibers associated with a motor unit contract maximally. This go or no-go characteristic is known as the *all or none law* of muscle contraction. The force produced by a particular muscle contraction is determined by the number of motor units *recruited* and *the force-producing potential of muscle mass within the motor unit.*

The number of muscle fibers in a single motor unit may vary from as few as 20, where fine, precise movement is required, to as many as 500 in large muscles of the thigh (10). Motor units with greater cross sectional area are generally capable of producing more force than those with less mass (25). The *gradation* of muscular force is accomplished by selective recruitment of the appropriate number and strength of motor units to do the required task.

Two other factors help explain the force generated by a muscle: *summation* and *synchronization*. If a threshold stimulus is applied to a motor unit, the muscle fibers contract. If, however, a second stimulus is applied before complete relaxation, the resulting contractile force is greater than that of the first contraction. This phenomenon is known as *summation*. At high frequencies of stimulation muscles enter a state of *tetanus*. The muscle tension achieved in tetanus is about twice that of a single twitch (10).

Synchronization is another factor helpful in understanding maximal muscle contraction. When extremely great muscular force is demanded, many motor units fire synchroniously and simultaneously. Unlike less demanding muscular contractions, which result in generally smooth movement, this synchronization may produce wavelike, jerky contractions of many skeletal muscles. These movements are most obvious when powerlifters attempt to lift very heavy weight, particularly when they attempt maximal deadlifts (25).

SOME BIOMECHANICS OF STRENGTH TRAINING

Muscle has only two functions: contraction (developing tension) and relaxation. Observable effects of muscle contraction and relaxation have been characterized as follows: *Isotonic contraction* is a muscle contraction that results in *observable movement*. The literal meaning of the word isotonic is "same tension," but very few, if any, movements made by the human body result in the same muscular tension throughout a range of motion. The changing length of the muscle and the changing mechanics of the lever system (skeletal system) make such an occurrence quite unlikely.

There are two subsets of isotonic contraction. The first is *concentric* contraction, which results when the force produced by the muscle is sufficient to overcome the resistance and the *muscle shortens*. Almost all skeletal muscles work in pairs set on opposite sides of joints, so when one muscle shortens (concentric contraction), another must lengthen. This lengthening is the second type of isotonic contraction and is called *eccentric* contraction. Eccentric contraction is a muscle contraction wherein the muscular force produced is insufficient to overcome the resistance and the *muscle lengthens*. Eccentric contraction is usually a controlled, voluntary movement, but it can be involuntary and potentially injurious, as in the case of a powerlifter collapsing under very heavy weight when attempting a maximum squat. All weight training exercises using gravity-resisted equipment are characterized by the same level of resistance in the concentric and eccentric phases.

Isometric or *static* contraction (meaning "same length') is muscle contraction that results in no observable movement. Isometric exercises, popularized during the 1950s by German researcher Theodore Hettinger (16) and others, have not been extensively practiced in strength training for many years.

STRENGTH CURVES AND ASSOCIATED EQUIPMENT DESIGN

The changing length of muscle and the changing mechanics of the lever system (skeletal system) in most ranges of motion of the human body produce force variations at different angles for each range of motion (ROM). These force variations plotted on a graph are referred to as *strength curves*. (See Figures 2–2 and 2–3.)

Figure 2–2
Elbow flexion strength at various angles in the range of motion. From C. F. Stiggins, Nautilus and free-weight training programs: A comparison of strength development at four angles in the range of motion, doctoral dissertation, Brigham Young University, 1978.

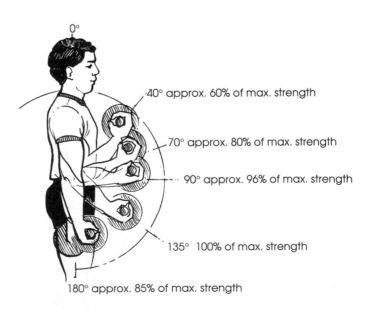

0°

40° approx. 60% of max. strength

70° approx. 80% of max. strength

90° approx. 96% of max. strength

135° 100% of max. strength

180° approx. 85% of max. strength

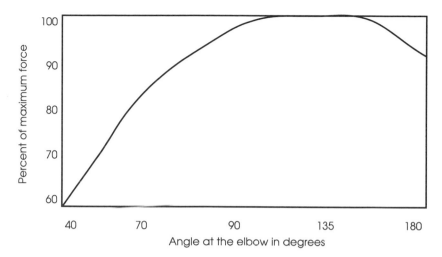

Figure 2–3
Force curve for elbow flexion. From C. F. Stiggins, Nautilus and free-weight training programs: A comparison of strength development at four angles in the range of motion, doctoral dissertation. Brigham Young University, 1978.

Variable Resistance

A commonly used method of determining the amount of resistance to use when weight training is to calculate a percentage of your one-repetition maximum (1RM) for each exercise in the program. Considering the strength curve concept, it becomes clear that a 1RM with a free bar (weight not attached to any machine) represents the strength a person has at the *weakest point* in the range of motion. If an individual could do a maximum curl with 100 pounds and wanted to do four sets at 70 percent of the 1RM, he or she would obviously use 70 pounds. Considering again the strength curve concept, the set with 70 pounds would offer 70 percent resistance only at the *weakest angle in the range of motion.* Other angles would be resisted at something less than 70 percent. An obvious question is associated with this phenomenon: Would it be any advantage to have 70 percent resistance at *all angles* in a range of movement, as opposed to 70 percent of maximum at only the weakest angle? A large percentage of the resistance machines marketed today claim to approximate this effect. *Variable resistance* machines are common in spas and weight rooms nationwide.

Nautilus *balanced variable resistance* weight training equipment was the first to introduce this concept. Universal *dynamic variable resistance* was next. Today many manufacturers produce such equipment. The resistance in Nautilus equipment is varied by a chain drive moving over cams of various shapes. (See Figure 2–4.) Resistance in Universal machines is varied through the use of a rolling (moving) weight-bearing point on a lever arm. As the weight-bearing roller moves further from the pivot point at the end of the lever, the resistance increases. (See Figure 2–5.)

Figure 2–4
Nautilus Omni Bicep Machine. Note
the crescent-shaped chain cam.
Variable resistance is achieved via
this cam.

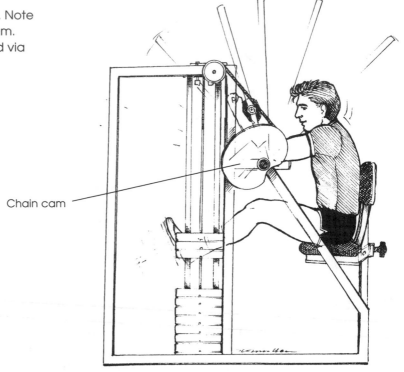

Chain cam

Figure 2–5
Universal Dynamic Variable Resistance Bench Press Station. As
handles are pressed upward,
weight-bearing point on lever arm
moves further from pivot point,
increasing resistance.

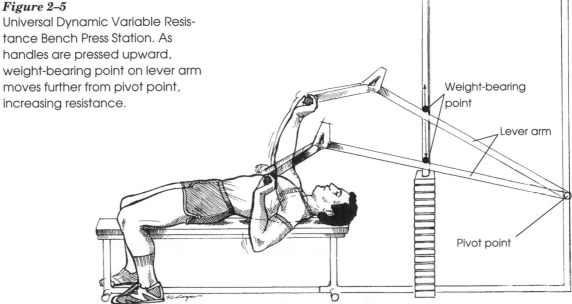

Weight-bearing
point

Lever arm

Pivot point

Figure 2–6
Mini Gym Squat
Thrust Station.
An isokinetic
machine.

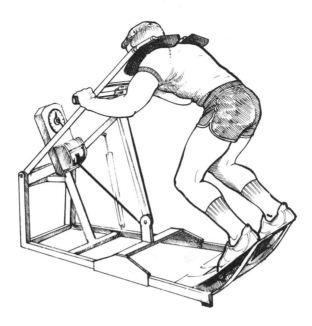

Isokinetic Resistance

The manufacturers of *isokinetic* equipment claim that their equipment accomodates the changing force potential within a ROM not unlike the variable resistance machines. However, in this case the variation in force is caused by variation in potential force within the human body, not the machine. The machine theoretically offers constant velocity movement no matter how much force is applied. Thus an exerciser must *apply the same degree of effort* throughout the ROM to produce the same relative degree of resistance at all angles. It is probably impossible for an exerciser to apply a particular *submaximal percentage of force* (e.g., 70 percent) at all angles in any range of motion. Therefore, when working on isokinetic equipment most exercisers simply apply *maximum force* throughout each range of motion. The force generated varies because the exerciser's potential to generate force varies.

Most isokinetic machines (see Figure 2–6) are equipped with adjustable speed mechanisms that allow them to be set from very slow to rather fast resistance speeds. Proponents of this type of exercise suggest that training at the higher velocities may be more specific to movements used in sports. Resistance in the eccentric phase of isokinetic exercise is negligible.

Because these machines are relatively safe (no weights to contend with if the exerciser decides to stop pulling or pushing) and the more expensive isokinetic equipment can produce graphs of strength curves, therapists and other sports medicine practitioners use these machines extensively in their work.

SPEED OF CONTRACTION WHILE WEIGHT TRAINING

In a concentric lift, the weight of the bar and the speed of movement possible are inversely related. In simple terms, lighter weights can be lifted faster than heavier weights. However, this relationship is hyperbolic, as opposed to linear. A fifty-pound bar cannot be moved twice as fast as a one hundred-pound bar.

A weight trainer might well ask, "How fast should I try to move a weight when weight training?" The best answer to that question is to move at a speed that seems comfortable and natural. If the weight is appropriate and if you do the correct number of repetitions, a comfortable speed will produce the desired effect.

Some coaches, particularly those involved in conditioning for sport, might suggest that a lifter move at a speed that is faster than that which seems comfortable or natural. The basis of this concept is the hope that by speeding up movement a person increases neuromuscular power. But at what combination of speed and resistance is human power maximized?

In a landmark study, Thorstensson (29) demonstrated that muscle power (force x distance/time) is maximized when the human body is resisted to the extent that it can only move at approximately 25 percent of its maximum potential velocity. At this velocity, power is optimal because force and velocity combine to produce the greatest human power output. At higher velocities with lighter loads, tension (muscular force) falls off, and with heavier loads velocity is reduced. The result is reduced power output.

Some teachers may suggest that you move at a purposefully slow speed when lifting weights. The Nautilus Corporation has been the major advocate of this concept. Moving at slow speeds supposedly ensures that muscles contract against the weight at each angle in the range of motion, as opposed to inertia moving a portion of the resistance.

The following points summarize what we know about speed of movement in weight training:

1. Well-planned and well-executed strength training can increase strength, speed, and power (power is essentially the ability to move a resistance quickly) (2, 4, 6, 14, 18, 20, 23, 24).
2. Relatively slow movements (normal speed) against high resistance (80–100 percent of 1RM) can produce gains in power superior to those produced by purposefully slow resisted movements (11, 22).
3. No evidence suggests that muscles hypertrophy more when lifters use purposefully slow movements as opposed to normal speed or faster movements when weight training. Hypertrophy seems more closely related to training intensity (weight), volume (no. of repetitions) and total load (total poundage lifted during a workout) than to speed of movement (23, 26).

PROGRESSIVE LOADING

One principle of strength training that is so obvious it might go without mention is that of progressive loading or overload (See Figure 2–7.) *Overload* is the term most frequently used to identify increases in resistance, but I prefer the words *progressive loading*.

All human beings intuitively know that if they are to improve at anything, they must tackle something a bit more difficult than that which they have mastered. This principle applies in any field of endeavor.

Success and consistent improvement in weight training is dependent on the amount of weight lifted, the number of repetitions, the rest between sets, the frequency of the workout, and other factors (nutrition, sleep, heredity, etc.). However, the grading of the resistance is very important. For relatively unconditioned people, resistance levels of 40 percent of maximum will cause strength improvement (12). For those who are extremely strong, lifting only 40 percent of their maximum would undoubtedly result in a strength loss. The level of resistance that weight trainers should normally use varies from 60 to 95 percent of the one-repetition maximum, depending on the desired result. The correct amount of resistance depends on the state of training of the individual and the particular program he or she is working on. (See Chapter Six for specific programs.)

When beginning a weight training program weight trainers should base their workout routines on their one-repetition maximums in each of the exercises. However, it may be somewhat uncomfortable or frightening for a beginning lifter to try one-repetition maximum lifts. One-repetition

Figure 2–7
Progressive loading

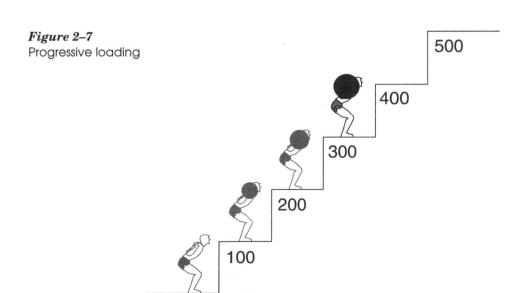

Table 2–2. Percentage of 1RM by repetitions

100% rep	97% 2 reps	94.5% 3 reps	89% 5 reps	85% 7 reps	83% 8 reps	75% 10 reps
100 lb	97 lb.	94 lb.	89 lb	85 lb.	83 lb.	76 lb.
120	117	113	107	102	100	91
135	131	126	120	115	112	103
150	146	142	134	128	125	114
170	165	161	151	145	141	129
190	185	180	169	162	158	144
210	204	198	187	179	174	160
230	212	217	205	196	191	175
250	243	236	223	213	208	190
270	262	254	240	230	224	205
290	282	274	258	247	241	220
310	301	293	276	264	257	236
330	321	312	294	281	274	251
350	340	330	312	298	291	266
370	360	350	329	315	307	281
390	380	367	347	331	324	296
410	399	387	365	348	340	312
430	418	406	383	366	357	327
450	437	425	400	382	374	342
470	457	444	418	400	390	357
500	486	473	445	425	425	380

Note: All weights are rounded to the nearest one pound.

maximum lifts can be approximated closely enough for developing most exercise routines by doing a set to failure and then predicting the 1RM using the Table 2–2, which has been developed from thousands of observations. The weights will not be precisely correct for each lift for every individual, but, they are close enough for a beginner to determine an initial weight to use for sets of ten or fewer repetitions.

SET-REPETITION COMBINATIONS FOR OPTIMAL STRENGTH AND FITNESS

Once researchers had determined that resistance exercise did indeed increase strength (5, 8), they wanted to find the combination of resistance levels, sets, and repetitions that produced strength the most quickly.

The first system touted to be the best was that of Dr. Thomas DeLorme, who did his early work in the 1940s. He developed a system based on a person's ten repetition maximum. He proposed a three-set routine consisting of one 10 rep. set at 1/2 the 10RM weight, the next 10 rep. set at 3/4 the 10RM weight, and the last 10 rep. set at the 10RM weight (8).

In a signal study, Dr. Richard A. Berger concluded that *three sets of the six repetition maximum* was the optimal workout for developing strength (4).

Michael Stone, Harold O'Bryant, and John Garhammer (27) have proposed a *periodization* or *cycling model* for improving strength, which has proven slightly superior to the 3x6 RM (3 sets of 6-repetition maximum) routine recommended by Dr. Berger (4).

Individuals interested in improving muscular fitness but not maximizing muscular strength may best go on a program of lifting moderate amounts of weight (60 to 70 percent of the 1RM) for 10 to 15 repetitions while reducing rest between sets to as little as 15 seconds.

A technique of doing partner-assisted repetitions *after reaching momentary muscular failure* is known as *forced repetitions*. This very demanding workout method usually involves doing a set number of partner assisted repetitions (3 to 5) or working until the assisting partner perceives that he is lifting 50 percent of the weight. No research has evaluated the effects of this extreme type of weight training. Those who use this technique are convinced that by so doing, hypertrophy is somewhat enhanced (7, 16). Table 2–3 can be helpful in designing various weight training/lifting programs.

Table 2–3. Work criteria for strength fitness, bodybuilding, and maximum strength weight-training/lifting programs.

Program objective	Sets	Reps	Approx. % of 1RM	Rest	Freq./ week	Days between workout
Strength fitness	3–4	8–12	70–80	1–2 min	3	1
Body building	4–8	8–20	65–85	30 sec	4–14	0
Max. Str.	3–6	1–6	80–100	3–6 min	2–4	1–3

(Strength fitness and bodybuilding are explained thoroughly in Chapter Four and high level strength training in Chapter Six. Conditioning for maximum strength would normally apply to athletes, Olympic lifters and powerlifters.)

SEQUENCING EXERCISES FOR BEST RESULTS

The principles that apply when sequencing a series of exercises are the following:

1. It is a good idea to do a warmup exercise at the beginning of the workout. A light, fast set of cleans or snatches serves this purpose well.
2. If you are a weightlifter or a weight trainer who does some multiple joint type exercises, you should put the large muscle-mass exercises first in your training program. Squats, cleans, deadlifts, and other exercises that tax most of the major moving muscles of the body should come prior to exercises that affect only the arms or the legs. The order of these large muscle-mass lifts might be changed periodically to ensure that each exercise is attempted in a relatively fatigue-free condition. Squats might be first on Monday, with deadlifts first on Wednesday, and cleans first on Friday.
3. Bodybuilders suggest that it is necessary to periodically change the exercises and/or the order of the exercises to get the best results. The best result usually implies the most muscular growth.

Other Methods of Enhancing Workout Results

Zero adaptation and *muscle confusion* have been suggested as a basis for periodically changing the exercises in a workout. The contention of bodybuilders (7, 16) is that after a few weeks on a particular exercise, the body has become so efficient that only the minimum number of motor units is stimulated when doing a particular lift. The exercise needs to be changed to cause the nervous system to send impulses to more or different motor units thereby stimulating more growth and/or strength. But, *no scientific evidence substantiates this concept.*

Variety is another good reason for changing exercises in a program. Workouts are usually more enjoyable when the exercises are periodically changed.

PERIODIZATION OR CYCLING

The concept of periodizing or cycling a weight training program, originally introduced by the Soviet L. Matveyev (17), has gained great favor among most weightlifters and others who train intensely. This process could be described as a controlled variation in the number of sets (volume), the weight lifted (intensity), and the number of workouts (frequency) over a prescribed period of time for the purpose of maximizing a person's strength or strength fitness at a chosen point in time. Periods could be as long as one year or more (macrocycle), a few months (mesocycle), or from one to four weeks (microcycle).

A beginning strength trainer can work on a variety of loosely structured programs and make progress. However, as weight trainers become stronger and more fit, they usually require more structured workout routines to reach higher levels of ability. Periodized strength training programs represent the most structured programs that have yet been developed.

Periodization is a controlled variation in the number of sets (volume), the weight lifted (intensity), and the number of workouts (frequency) over a prescribed period of time for the purpose of maximizing a person's strength or strength fitness at a point in time.

General Adaptation Syndrome (GAS)

This concept of cycling or periodizing a training program is derived from the theory of the *General Adaptation Syndrome (GAS)* formulated by Dr. Hans Selye (19). (See Figure 2–8.) GAS explains the body's response to stressors (heat, emotion, germs, exercise, etc.) which demand that the body adjust to maintain homeostasis (normal balance of body functions and processes).

There are three phases in the GAS. All organisms exhibit this triphase response when exposed to stressors.

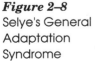

Figure 2–8
Selye's General
Adaptation
Syndrome

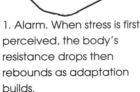

Normal | Level of Resistance

1. Alarm. When stress is first perceived, the body's resistance drops then rebounds as adaptation builds.

2. Adaptation. As stress continues resistance rises above normal (stress within adaptation limits).

3. Exhaustion. After prolonged exposure to stress, adaptation energy is exhausted and resistance drops. Death results if stress continues.

1. Alarm. The first phase of GAS, the body recognizes and prepares to cope with a new stimulus. Defense mechanisms are activated. There is increased pulse rate, redistribution of blood, and elevated blood sugar.
2. Adaptation. The *adaptation* phase follows and corresponds to a time during which an individual makes reasonable improvement in his or her conditioning. The alarm stage is overcome, and the body adapts to the stress by improving its capacity to function.
3. Exhaustion. If the stimulus is too strong or too long, this third stage is reached. Individuals who reach the third stage are overtrained. The time an organism will be in each phase depends on the stimulus.

The implications are obvious for any weight trainer. Train with intensity but don't overtrain. How does one determine if he or she is overtraining? By observing the results of a training period and of course, how one generally feels. Overtraining will result in decreased effectiveness and a stale, down feeling.

Table 2–4 presents the general concepts of periodization: By properly using this model, strength trainers can design programs that facilitate con-

Table 2–4 Theoretical model of strength training derived from Matveyev's periodization model

	Preparation Strength[1] Foundation	Transition-1 Basic Strength	Strength & Power	Competition Peaking or Maintenance	Transition-2 AR[3]
Sets	3-5	3-5	3-5	1-3	
Reps	8-20	2-6	2-4	1-3	
Days/wk	3-4	3-5	3-6	1-5	
Times/day	1-3	1-3	1-2	1	
Intensity cycle (wks)[2]	2-3/1	2-4/1	1-3/1	2-10	1-3
Intensity level	Low	High	High	Very high	
Volume	High	Mod.	Low	Very low	

[1] The original model refers to this phase as the *hypertrophy* phase.

[2] The intensity cycle 2-3/1 means 2 or 3 weeks of heavy work followed by 1 light week.

[3] AR = Active Rest. Very little or no lifting; engage in other activity.

Source: From M. H. Stone, H. O'Bryant, J. Garhammer, et al., 1982. A theoretical model of strength training, *National Strength and Conditioning Association Journal* 3–5:36–39.

ditioning without overtraining. (See the chapters on strength fitness and high-level strength training for examples of periodized workout routines.)

DELAYED MUSCLE SORENESS (DMS)

When a person begins an exercise program, soreness in the muscles usually results in from twelve to forty-eight hours after the exercise bout. The cause of this muscle soreness is not fully understood. However, some research on the issue is interesting to consider. Talag studied the relationship of muscle soreness to concentric, eccentric, and isometric contractions. She found that the muscles of the group trained solely with eccentric contractions became extremely sore, while the concentrically and isometrically trained groups experienced very little muscle soreness. This suggests that eccentric contractions contribute significantly to muscle soreness after exercise (28).

deVries's spasm theory of delayed muscle soreness suggests that exercise brings about localized muscle ischemia (deficiency of blood); this ischemia causes pain, which generates increased reflex motor activity. Greater motor activity in turn creates higher local muscle tension, which results in even greater muscle ischemia. deVries's research suggests that static muscle stretching helps prevent and relieve soreness (9).

Abraham found muscle soreness to correlate with the appearance of myoglobin in the urine. Myoglobinuria is a marker of muscle fiber trauma that is characteristic of all strenuous work, independent of muscle soreness. Abraham also considered hydroxyproline excretion, which indicates connective tissue breakdown. He found a significant correlation between the day of maximal hydroxyproline excretion and the day when subjects experienced their greatest soreness (1).

Bansil et al., have reported that prostaglandins play a role in delayed muscle soreness. Prostaglandins are "hormones" formed from unsaturated fatty acids. It is known that certain prostaglandins (PGE) facilitate the formation of inflammatory substances such as histamine and bradykinin. Bansil et al., therefore, suggest that delayed muscle soreness is an inflammatory response brought about by synthesis of adequate amounts of PGE twelve to thirty-six hours after exercise (3).

This evidence suggests that when we are in the first week or two of an exercise program, or when we change from one activity to another, deVries's spasm theory of motor activity and resulting ischemia are triggered. Additionally, for some reason as yet unexplained, the eccentric movements we make during the initial stages of exercise cause breakdown of both muscle fibers and connective tissue. This breakdown possibly results in prostaglandin formation, which precipitates the release of other inflammatory agents within the body. However, further research needs to be done to substantiate these postulates.

REST OR RECOVERY BETWEEN SETS AND EXERCISES

The time it takes to rest and recover between sets or exercises depends on many factors. Frequently the time is determined by the length of discussions with training partners or others, as opposed to a necessary recovery of physical working capacity (PWC).

Bodybuilders often try to move from set to set with as little as fifteen to thirty seconds of recovery time. Bodybuilders, who usually work at moderate resistance levels, believe that they get a much better pump—the major objective of their workout—by resting only a few seconds between sets. The most logical explanation for this ability to repeat strenuous sets without longer recovery time is that the set does not totally deplete the energy stores of the muscle and/or the muscle has been conditioned so that energy stores are rapidly replenished.

Powerlifters and Olympic-style lifters often rest three to five minutes or more between sets. Their objective is to become stronger and lift heavier weight. The volume of musculature required for doing most of the power or Olympic lifts is much greater than that required for most bodybuilding exercises. The greater muscle mass undoubtedly requires more time for energy restoration.

The ATP-CP energy system (phosphogens) is the energy system of choice when lifting heavy weights only a few repetitions. Phosphogen stores provide large amounts of energy for short periods of time. Ten seconds of maximal exercise would essentially deplete a muscle's available phosphogen stores; however, within 2 1/2 to 3 minutes these stores would be 99 percent replenished (26).

In summary, weight trainers interested in a muscle pump should try to try to reduce rest intervals to one minute or less. Recovery from upper body exercises usually requires less time than recovery from lower body exercises. Those interested in maximizing strength should use rest intervals of three minutes or more. The person who is interested in strength fitness should rest no more than two minutes between sets.

ERGOGENIC AIDS

Since the beginning of competitive sport, man has sought an edge over his opponent. Techniques or substances that might improve performance beyond levels normally anticipated or expected from orthodox training techniques have been the object of a never-ending search. There are many potential ergogenic aids.

In his definitive book *Ergogenic Aids in Sport,* Melvin Williams classifies ergogenic aids into five categories: nutritional, pharmacological, physiological, psychological, and mechanical (31). Indeed, anything that might aid athletic performance could be classified as an ergogenic aid. An erg is a measure of energy; *genic* is derived from genesis, which means "giving rise to." Therefore ergogenic means that which gives rise to, or assists in, energy production. Athletes and others regularly use ergogenic aids; that is, training programs, vitamins, energy supplying drinks, oxygen breathing, and weight training. Most ergogenic aids have been accepted by the athletic world and the public as being ethical to use. However, the public has cried out against the use of performance enhancing pharmacological substances (drugs such as amphetamines, cocaine, and anabolic steroids) and blood doping (physiological category). Blood doping is the practice of removing blood from your system, storing it, training for a period of time, then reinjecting the blood prior to an important contest. The extra number of red blood cells gives an athlete an increased oxygen-carrying capacity.

Amphetamines and other "uppers" leave an easily detected physiological imprint, and their use is supposedly not widespread. The use of anabolic steroids, on the other hand, has developed into a major international problem.

Anabolic Steroids

Anabolic steroid use has cast a shadow over athletic and other strength-building pursuits that exceeds even the negative impact of muscle boundness rampant in the 1940s and 1950s. These drugs are generally synthetic derivatives of the male hormone testosterone. Testosterone is the male sex hormone that is largely responsible for increases in muscular size in males. Most women produce only small amounts of this hormone; therefore they do not have large muscles. Anabolic steroids increase the nitrogen content of the muscle cell, which causes an increase in protein synthesis, which increases muscular size and strength.

They were first introduced to athletes in the United States by a physician and weightlifter, Dr. John Ziegler. Dr. Ziegler was appointed as the team physician for U.S. weightlifters at the world championships of 1954 in Vienna, Austria. While on that trip he discovered the use of testosterone among Soviet weightlifters. He and some close associates tried testosterone and found that it helped to improve their strength. Dr. Ziegler then worked with a pharmaceutical company to develop Dianabol (methandrostenolone) in the late 1950s. He administered Dianabol to some of the athletes training at the York Barbell Club and the rage began (30, 32). Seeing the dangerous side effects of this new drug Dr. Ziegler tried to stop its use, but it was too late.

A few of the more well-known anabolic agents are Dianabol, Winstrol, Durabolin 50, Decadurabolin, and Nilavar. Human growth hormone (HGH) or Somatotropin could be added to the list today. By 1989 the use of anabolic steroids had reached massive, worldwide proportions.

Anabolic steroid use has cast a shadow of question over athletic pursuits that exceeds even the negative impact of muscle boundness rampant in the 1940s and 1950s.

For some time after anabolic steroids were introduced, researchers and others suggested that such drugs did not enhance athletic performance. Athletes simply did not agree. As they used the drugs performances requiring high levels of strength and quickness improved. Not only did strength increase but there was a concomitant gain in muscle mass. Bodybuilders were overjoyed.

Although researchers have suggested for some years now that the drugs are not effective, an ever-increasing number of athletes and bodybuilders exhibit through their performances and testimonials the positive effects of these drugs. How much do anabolic steroids help performance? There is no definitive answer. My experience leads me to believe that the degree of effect for a population of athletes would approximate a normal curve, most users noticing some enhancement of strength/power, some not being aware of any, and others realizing very significant gains. Based on my observations over the past twenty-five years it is not unreasonable to suggest that performances may be increased from 3 to 10 percent over nonsteroid use capabilities.

Based on the author's observations over the past twenty-five years it is not unreasonable to suggest that steroid aided performances may be increased from 3 to 10 percent over drug-free efforts.

Refreshingly, and thankfully, there is a small group of people of some credibility—coaches and a very small number of athletes—who suggest that anabolic steroids are not necessary to very high level (world class), power-type athletic performance. If only that were true! If what they profess were true, the problems these drugs create would not exist. A much,

much larger number of credible people cannot refute what they see as evidence that anabolic steroids do indeed increase performance potential.

There is a small group of people of some credibility who, as of 1990, suggests that anabolic steroids are not necessary to achieve very high level (world class), power-type athletic performance. There are much larger numbers of credible individuals who believe otherwise.

After a number of years of struggling with what to do about the anabolic steroid problem, sports governing bodies have begun to take action to slow, if not stop, the use of these drugs. The International Olympic Committee banned the drugs in 1972. Scandinavian countries and Great Britain started punitive drug testing during the late 1970s, and the United States joined the effort at the Olympic Trials of 1984. The NCAA mounted a drug testing program in 1986, specifically in response to the growing use of anabolic steroids.

Most athletes and some nations (the Soviet Union and East Germany) have not responded to these testing programs as officials had hoped. Rather than giving up the use of these performance-aiding substances, many athletes have done everything possible to beat the tests. For several years the USSR and the GDR have researched the effects of anabolic steroids on their athletes (21). But athletes from the United States have been taking the drugs illicitly and secretly, with no coordinated effort to evaluate the physiological or psychological effects they produce.

The pressure to win, or at least to be competitive, and the belief that using anabolic steroids and other drugs is necessary to achieve these goals, plus the confidence that there is a way to avoid getting caught are more powerful in the minds of most athletes than concern about side effects and drug tests. Sports governing bodies have become drug enforcement agencies; and the athletes, who have been frequently looked on as models to emulate in our society, are considered drug-taking suspects similar to heroine or cocaine addicts.

Resources sorely needed for athletic research and development are being diverted to medical institutions to pay for drug testing. Millions of dollars have been spent and are being spent on testing athletes for the illicit use of drugs. In my opinion, the testing programs are not stopping the use of performance-aiding drugs, but they are draining much-needed resources from other important programs.

Because of societal pressure to stop the use of these drugs random testing measures have been instituted by at least one national governing body. The Athletics Congress (TAC, the National Track and Field governing body) began random drug testing in October of 1989.

> Sports governing bodies have become drug enforcement agencies and athletes, who have been frequently looked on as models to emulate in our society, are considered drug-taking suspects similar to heroine or cocaine addicts.

Enforcement personnel appearing at the door of a suspect and demanding either a blood or urine sample is totalitarian and an invasion of privacy. This should be considered in only the most extreme situations. Testing at competitions seems to be more within acceptable limits to a free society. However, random, punitive testing may be the only way to rid sports of the current epidemic.

Potential Dangers—Side Effects of Anabolic Steroids. A great deal has been written about the potential problems associated with anabolic steroid use. It must be accepted that use of these drugs does produce undesirable side effects. Some of these are as follows:

> Liver damage. The most commonly documented side effects are changes in liver function. Oral anabolics produce more problems than injectables.
> Dramatic reduction of high density lipoprotein (HDL-C) and an increase in low density lipoproteins (LDL-C). These two conditions contribute to increased risk of cardiovascular disease.
> Increased irritability (increased aggressiveness).
> Impaired pituitary and thyroid function.
> Increase in blood pressure or nervous tension.
> Disorders of the prostate gland.
> Changes in reproductive systems (testicular atrophy).
> Sex drive fluctuations (increased then decreased).
> Increased body and facial hair; thinning of hair on scalp.
> Acne, skin rash.
> Gynecomastia (development of breastlike tissue in males), sore nipples.
> Headaches, dizziness, nose bleeds, drowsiness.
> Muscle cramps and spasms.

Women who use anabolics with the hope of increasing their muscularity or performance potential face most of the side effects listed above plus some others, as follows:

> Menstrual irregularities.
> Deepening of the voice (nonreversible).

Clitoral enlargement.

Increased collagen (the fibrous component of connective tissue).

Increased body and facial hair (nonreversible).

In all sports the use of anabolic steroids and all other performance-enhancing drugs must be stopped. They threaten athletes and they threaten the institution of sport generally. We must carefully consider the various means by which drug use might be eradicated. Decisions may be difficult, but decisions need to be made and actions taken to make sport drug-free.

The sports institutions face a grave situation in the United States. We must stop the use of performance aiding drugs and preserve sport as a positive, character-building experience for all who take part.

It is my opinion, after years of closely associating with many athletes, that this dilemma will not be resolved within the near future.

REFERENCES

1. Abraham, W. M. 1979. Exercise induced muscle soreness. *Physician and Sports Medicine* 7: 57–60.
2. Anderson, T., and J. T. Kearney. 1982. Effects of three resistance training programs on muscular strength and absolute and relative endurance. *Research Quarterly for Exercise and Sport* 53: 1–7.
3. Bansil, C. K., G. D. Wilson, and M. H. Stone. 1985. Role of prostaglandins E and F2 alpha in exercise-induced delayed muscle soreness (abstract). *Medicine and Science in Sport and Exercise* 17: 276.
4. Berger, R. A. 1963. Comparison of the effect of three weight training programs on strength. *Research Quarterly*. 34: 396–398.
5. Capen, E. K. 1950. The effect of systematic weight training on power, strength, and endurance. *Research Quarterly* 31: 83–93
6. Clark, D. H., and F. M. Henry. 1961. Neuromotor specificity and increase speed from strength development. *Research Quarterly* 32: 315–325.
7. Curtis S. 1979. Personal communication, February.
8. DeLorme, T. L., and A. L. Watkins. 1948. Techniques of progressive resistance exercise. *Archives of Physical Medicine* 29: 263.
9. deVries, H. A. 1974. *Physiology of Exercise for Physical Education and Athletes*, 2nd ed. Dubuque, Iowa: Wm. C. Brown.
10. Fox, E. L., and D. K. Mathews. 1981. *The Physiological Basis of Physical Education and Athletics,* 3rd ed. Philadelphia: Saunders.
11. Garhammer, J. 1979. Power production by Olympic weightlifters. *Medicine and Science in Sports and Exercise* 12: 54–60.
12. Gettman, L. R., and Pollock, M. L. 1981. Circuit weight training: A critical review of physiological benefits. *Physician and Sports Medicine* 9: 1.
13. Guyton, A. C. 1986. *Textbook of Medical Physiology,* 7th ed. Philadelphia: Saunders.
14. Hakkinen, K., and P. Komi. 1982. Alterations of mechanical characteristics of human skeletal muscle during strength training. *European Journal of Applied Physiology* 50: 161–172

15. Hettinger, T., M. D. 1961. *The Physiology of Strength.* Springfield Ill.: Charles C. Thomas.

16. Jenkins, B. 1983. Personal communication, January.

17. Matveyev, L. 1981. *Fundamentals of Sport Learning* (trans. Albert P. Zdornykh). Moscow: Progress Publishers.

18. Rasch, P. J. 1982. *Weight Training,* 4th ed. Dubuque, Iowa: Wm. C. Brown.

19. Selye, H. 1956. *The Stress of Life* New York: Lippincott.

20. Schmidbleicher, D., and G. Haralombie. 1981. Changes in contractile properties of muscle after strength training in man. *European Journal of Applied Physiology* 46: 221–228.

21. Schmidt, W. 1988. Personal communication, April.

22. Smith, L. E., and L. D. Whitley, 1965. Influence of strengthening exercise on speed of limb movement. *Archives of Physical Medicine and Rehabilitation* 46: 772–777.

23. Silvester, L. J. 1976. A comparison of the effect of variable resistance and free-weight training programs on muscular strength, vertical jump, and thigh circumference. Doctoral dissertation, Brigham Young University, Provo, Utah.

24. Smith, L. E., and L. D. Whitley. 1966. Influence of three different training programs on strength and speed of limb movement. *Research Quarterly* 37: 132–142.

25. Stiggins, C. F. 1978. Nautilus and free-weight training programs: A comparison of strength development at four angles in the range of motion. Masters thesis, Brigham Young University, Provo, Utah.

26. Stone M. H. and H. O'Bryant. 1987. *Weight Training a Scientific Approach.* Minneapolis: Bellwether Press.

27. Stone, M. H., H. O'Bryant, J. Garhammer, et al., 1982. A theoretical model of strength training. *National Strength and Conditioning Association Journal* 35: 36–39.

28. Talag, T. S. 1973. Residual muscle soreness as influenced by concentric, eccentric, and static contractions. *Research Quarterly* 44: 458–469

29. Thorstensson, A. 1976. Muscle strength, fiber types, and enzymes in man. *Acta Physiologica Scandanavica: Supplementum* 443.

30. Todd, T. 1983. The steroid predicament. *Sports Illustrated* 59: 62–66.

31. Williams, M. H., ed. 1980. *Ergogenic Aids in Sport.* Champaign, Ill.: Human Kinetics.

32. Windsor, R. E., and D. Dumitu. 1988. Anabolic steroid use by athletes: How serious are the health hazards? *Postgraduate Medicine* 15(4): 37–38, 41–43, 47–49.

CHAPTER THREE

Weight Training and Physical Fitness

*T*o what extent do you enjoy life? Is life challenging and enjoyable, or is it a series of stressful events that don't turn out very well? We might all benefit from asking ourselves those questions.

To get the most out of life we must be physically fit. Our bodies should enable us to enjoy physical activity and doing our daily tasks without breaking down or becoming overly tired. It would be good if they also helped us feel confident about ourselves. For some of us a physically fit body is a natural consequence of the life we live.

One of the important requirements for us if we are to get the most out of life is to have a physically fit body.

Observe a group of children for a day. You will see them run, jump, roll around, laugh, argue, perhaps fight, and play with a great sense of purpose. Generally, they are in constant motion. They move about incessantly because that is what they instinctively enjoy doing. It is really what they must do if they are to develop normally. At some point you would see them sleep. They sleep the deep, refreshing sleep of physically tired, innocent children. Fitness for children is normal if they are allowed freedom to follow their instincts.

Movement for children is important for many reasons, not just for physical development. Children's physical fitness relates to their mental achievement. H. Harrison Clarke, editor of the *Physical Fitness Research Digest*, concluded an extensive review of articles related to mental achievement and fitness by saying, "It may be contended that a person's general learning potential for a given level of intelligence increases or decreases in accordance with his degree of physical fitness" (5). Unless the activity of children is restricted by parents, environment (areas without adequate opportunity for movement), or disability, children naturally engage in adequate activity to be quite physically fit.

As we mature we must "act more like adults," and adults in the United States are characteristically sedentary (19). Is life best lived in a sedentary manner? Despite those who say that when they get an urge to exercise they lie down until the urge passes, very few of us, if any, would agree that life is best lived in an armchair.

SOME CULTURAL REASONS FOR UNFIT AMERICANS

The Industrial Revolution and the mechanization and modernization of our world have wonderfully and yet somewhat insidiously changed our lives. The insidiousness of this change that is the concern of this book, is the *decrease in physical activity resulting from the myriad of time- and work-saving devices that have been invented.* Wonderful they are, because they give us more freedom and efficiency than ever before. They accomplish tasks in minutes with little effort that formerly took hours or even days of demanding physical work. The movement from rural to an urban society eliminated the requirement to do physical work for a large percentage of our society. Even in rural areas physical work demands have been greatly reduced.

Consider plowing, planting, and harvesting a field. Tractors and other machinery have made these processes relatively easy. Washing clothes and washing dishes? The machines that do these tasks today no longer require us to wring and rinse. Preparing a meal? This can still take time and work, but often it does not. Mowing the lawn? Compare hand-pushed, reel-type mowers to self-propelled or riding mowers. Getting from our homes to the local stores? Compare walking or riding a horse or bicycle to driving an automobile.

Devices which save time and reduce physical labor are particularly evident in the work place. We are living in a highly mechanized and com-

Figure 3-1 Should you join a fitness center?

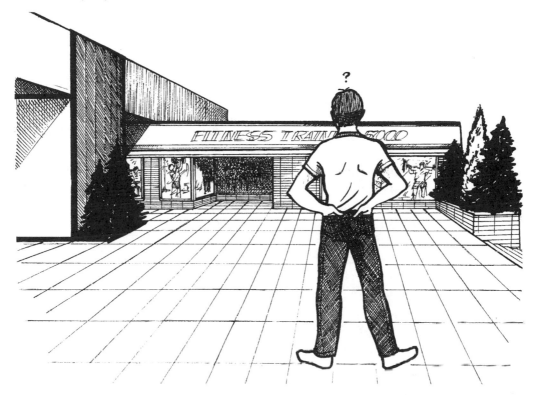

puterized society, but we still have frontier bodies that need some vigorous physical work!

A work day usually lacking in physical activity, and life facilitated by computers, cars, labor-saving devices, and the fast food industry, and fraught with urban overcrowding have combined to produce a United States society of generally overweight, overstressed citizens who lack physical fitness.

The fast food industry has contributed to our dilemma by creating food items that are fast, tasty, and convenient, with a caloric composition of at least 40 percent fat. A Big Mac counts out at a hefty 53 percent fat. Many of us who are employed in professions requiring little physical movement have become underexercised and overweight. These conditions can have such a negative effect on our health and self-esteem that we often don't feel good about getting out and doing anything physical, even though we need it. Exercise can become physically painful, or more frequently, just too embarrassing.

HYPOKINETIC DISEASE

When we stop exercising for whatever reason we become hypokinetic. *Hypo* means too little or less than normal, and *kinetic* refers to motion and the energy associated with that motion. In other words, too little energy expenditure! Millions of Americans have physical debilities resulting from hypokinetic lifestyles. If a person becomes hypokinetic, the following difficulties may ultimately result: lethargy, deterioration of strength, atrophy of muscle, deterioration of bone, poor appetite, inability to sleep well (insomnia), constipation, nervousness, hyperactivity (in children), and a whole host of associated problems (7, 17).

We are all thankful for the many marvelous inventions that save us time and effort, but we should seek the knowledge and wisdom to deal with these inventions and the conditions they create. We know all of us need to participate in an exercise program so we can function at our best both physically and mentally (5, 7).

EXERCISE AND FITNESS

What is a physically fit body? The basic components of fitness are cardiorespiratory fitness, strength, muscular power, muscular endurance, flexibility, and body composition (neither overly fat nor overly thin). Individuals interested in developing or maintaining a reasonable level of fitness should devote some attention to each of these components during exercise periods. How much and what type of exercise does a normal person need to maintain a healthy, fit body? This question can be answered by considering what the American College of Sports Medicine (ACSM) has said about a "well rounded" exercise program. The ACSM modified its exercise guidelines in 1990 for the first time in twelve years. The purpose of the modification was to include a recommendation for "resistance" training.

The ACSM Exercise Recommendations

ACSM recommended aerobic training

1. Mode of activity (What kind?): Any activity that uses large muscle groups, that can be maintained continuously, and that is rhythmical and aerobic in nature—e.g., walking, hiking, jogging, running,

swimming, skating, bicycling, rowing, cross-country skiing, rope skipping, and various endurance games.

2. Frequency of exercise (How often?): three to five days per week.
3. Intensity of training (How hard?): 60–90 percent of maximal heart rate reserve, or 50–85 percent of maximal oxygen uptake (VO_2 max.)
4. Duration of training (How long?): 15–60 minutes of continuous aerobic activity. Duration depends on intensity of the activity: lower intensity activity should be conducted over a longer period of time. Because "total fitness" is more readily attained in longer duration programs, and because hazards and compliance problems are associated with high intensity activity, lower to moderate intensity activity of longer duration is recommended for the nonathletic adult (2).

ACSM recommended resistance training

1. Engage in resistance training at least twice per week.
2. Your workout routine should include a minimum of eight to ten exercises, exercises that affect all of the major muscle groups of the body.
3. Exercise at a moderate intensity level; do not try to lift weight that is too heavy.
4. You should do at least one set in each exercise with momentary muscular failure occurring somewhere between eight and twelve repetitions.

It is interesting to note that heart rates achieved during circuit weight training are high enough (60–90 percent of max. heart rate reserve) to be considered adequate for a cardiorespiratory endurance program, but for some reason oxygen uptake (VO_2) values (defined below) are less than 50 percent of the maximal level (12, 13). Weight training is very effective in improving strength and muscular power (7, 12, 18, 19). Certain routines can enhance muscular endurance and flexibility (12, 18, 19). However, most weight training programs simply do not require enough oxygen to give our oxygen supplying mechanisms a good workout (12, 13). Therefore, weight training programs should be supplemented with an aerobic workout at least three times per week.

DO WHAT YOU ENJOY

How should you go about setting up an exercise program to assure that you include all of the components of fitness? One example of a good fitness program would be: 30 minutes of basketball (aerobic, muscular endurance and muscular power) followed by 30 minutes of weight training (muscular strength, muscular power, and muscular endurance) and another 10–15 minutes of stretching (flexibility); and a 30–minute jog (aerobic) on days when you don't play basketball. But you should do something you enjoy doing.

An hour of basketball or tennis with friends three times per week may not include attention to all components of fitness, but it is far superior to starting and then quitting the other activities. Of course, I hope that on those days when you cannot arrange something fun with your friends you have enough discipline to do something else to ensure your continued good health and fitness.

Do something you enjoy doing. A fun game of basketball or racquetball with friends three times per week is far superior to designing a thorough fitness workout then quitting after a few weeks.

AEROBIC FITNESS

Some years ago Dr. Kenneth Cooper, of the Aerobics Institute in Dallas, Texas, did research for the Air Force on exercise. He was charged to develop a field test of fitness and then use it to measure the fitness of Air Force personnel. To identify fitness categories or levels, he tested thousands of men. Dr. Cooper ultimately developed a test that has proven very popular. In this test, fitness categories are determined by how fast a person runs or jogs one and one-half miles. The age-adjusted fitness categories are: superior, excellent, good, fair, poor, and very poor (6). A male thirteen to nineteen years of age who ran 1.5 miles between 8:37 and 9:40 would be in the excellent category for cardiovascular fitness. A female in the same age category would need to run between 11:50 and 12:29 to be in the same excellent category (6).

The results of Dr. Cooper's work and his ideas about fitness are found in his books *Aerobics* and *The Aerobics Way*. Dr. Cooper's influence in the field of fitness is without parallel. As a result of his work and the "catching on" of his ideas, which are and have been used by hundreds of teachers and writers, millions of people have engaged in aerobic exercise programs.

Aerobic exercise essentially means exercising at a moderate work rate that allows the body to supply oxygen to the working tissues at the same rate that oxygen is being used to produce energy. When we refer to a person's aerobic power we generally refer to their maximum oxygen uptake (VO_2 max.), or the maximum ability of the body to deliver and use or take up oxygen in the working muscles.

Aerobic exercise has two important effects on our bodies. First, our engines (heart, lungs) are appropriately challenged. This simply means they are worked at a moderate rate over a reasonable period of time (15 minutes or more). The rate of improvement and the degree of such improvement are determined generally by the exercise program, our heredity, and our age. The second important effect of aerobic exercise is its role in burning fat, or as we often refer to it, its role in weight control. Make no mistake about it, Americans of the 1990s eat better and live longer than any of their predecessors, but we do have some problems with what we eat and the resultant adiposity (fat). Let us consider how to easily set up an aerobic exercise program.

Developing an Aerobic Fitness Program

To help you set up your own aerobics program, let us consider a sample program for a twenty-two-year-old female who has a resting heart rate (RHR) of 66 beats per minute (b/min).

Take your RHR by putting your first two fingers either on the radial artery on the thumb side of your wrist (See Figure 3–2) or on the carotid artery on either side of your neck (See Figure 3–3). Taking an accurate pulse rate in a resting state usually requires sensitivity and a little prac-

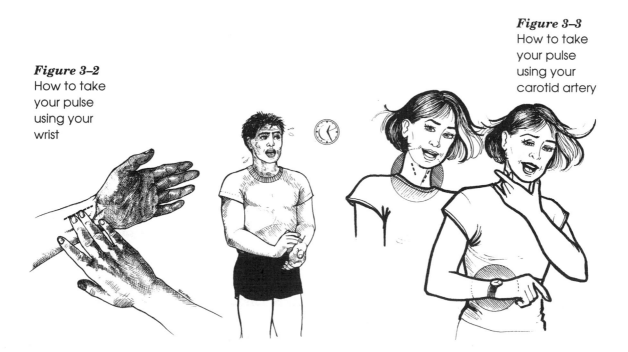

Figure 3–3
How to take
your pulse
using your
carotid artery

Figure 3–2
How to take
your pulse
using your
wrist

tice. Count the heart rate for 10 seconds, counting the first count as zero (zero, one, two, etc.), then multiply the result by 6 to get the one-minute rate.

Karvonen and his associates (15) devised a way of estimating maximum heart rate and from that an associated system of controlling the intensity of aerobic exercise. First, to estimate our subject's maximum heart rate (MHR) we subtract her age from 220. Her estimated MHR would be 198. Next we need to determine the range of exercise intensity for her program. Karvonen's system uses the following formula to determine the training heart rate range (THRR):

$$THRR = .6 \text{ to } .9 \text{ of } (MHR - RHR) + RHR$$

The following calculations would then determine the THRR for our subject:

$$THRR = .6 \text{ to } .9 \text{ of } (MHR = 198 - RHR = 66) + 66$$
$$THRR = .6 \text{ to } .9 \text{ of } (132) + 66$$
$$THRR = (79 \text{ to } 119) + 66$$
$$THRR = 145 - 185 \text{ b/min}$$

Considering the American College of Sports Medicine (ACSM) guidelines, then, our subject should engage in a continuous aerobic exercise three times per week for at least 15 minutes each session, with her heart ranging between 145 and 185 b/min. Please remember that you should engage in an aerobic activity you find enjoyable! Anyone starting an exercise program would probably be most comfortable starting at the low end of the range and gradually progressing.

➤ *What would you include in a total fitness program? Design a total fitness program for one week that could be used each week for a year.*

SOME SOCIETAL CONDITIONS AND NATIONAL HEALTH

Our information-based society and the fast-food industry referred to earlier have taken their toll on the health and vigor of a large portion of our population. Most of our diets have increased in fat content while our exercise or physical work requirements have diminished to almost zero.

One of the great struggles in the history of the human race has been to throw off the burden of physical work. Landowners, masters, and kings throughout history were admired because of their lives of ease. For most of the population prior to 1900, life required difficult and demanding physical labor. Today, many if not most United States citizens are not required to engage in physical work to earn their livelihood. Ironically, this "freedom from physical labor" has been found to be a debilitating and even deadly when combined with a diet high in saturated fat. You might conclude that you can not win, but you really can. Just read on.

Many of the citizens living in the United States have arrived at what could be considered a life of relative ease. Surprisingly, this life has been found to be potentially debilitating and even deadly when combined with a diet high in saturated fat.

Another condition in the United States and some other parts of the world is perhaps unique in the history of humanity: an overabundance of food. We have the capacity to purchase and consume much more food than we need to function. Many of us, perhaps quite naturally, eat more than we should. I say "quite naturally" because most animals, if given large amounts of food, will eat it. Perhaps we do so because of some primeval urge to eat up in order to hedge against the times when food will be in short supply, or perhaps we do so simply because eating is pleasurable. Perhaps we overeat because when we worked and played as youth we could eat food and burn the calories, but as we matured our work or exercise rate decreased but our appetites remained the same. Or perhaps we become overweight not because we eat more food but because our food contains more calories, particularly fat calories. Suffice it to say that many of us find ourselves somewhat overweight, wondering how we got there and thinking we might be well advised to lose a few pounds. We are concerned both about appearance and good health.

This situation in the United States has given rise to a multimillion-dollar industry that is consistently growing. Nutri/System, New Shape Center, Weight Loss Clinic, Weight Watchers, and Diet Center are some of the corporations that make it their business to help Americans with weight problems. Many smaller businesses such as spas and health clubs have similar purposes. Millions of us are overweight and many businesses have been established to help us lose body fat, for a price. Weight loss in America is big business.

We have discovered that human beings need some *vigorous* work to function properly. We now refer to such work as *exercise,* partly because of the social stigma associated with physical work (only the lower classes do such work). Vigorous exercise could be defined as exercise at a rate that causes a person to break into a sweat. Because of the very positive effects that appropriate aerobic exercise has on the cardiovascular system of the body, and the further positive effect of burning fat calories, such exercise is thought to be quite beneficial. Indeed, it is good for all of us to engage in a consistent aerobic exercise program to keep ourselves totally fit. Clearly, walking, jogging, swimming, and cross-country skiing are good aerobic activities. But what about weight training?

WEIGHT TRAINING AND AEROBIC CAPACITY

Does weight training produce any aerobic changes? In a thorough review of the literature, Gettman and Pollack concluded that circuit weight training (CWT) can improve cardiorespiratory endurance, body composition, and strength, but sessions must last 25 to 30 minutes (12). The studies Gettman and Pollack reviewed showed about a 5 percent increase in aerobic capacity, compared to 15 to 25 percent improvement for other forms of aerobic exercise.

Weight training circuits are usually designed to exercise all of the major muscle groups of the body. They can be either free weights, machines, or both. Resistance levels are moderate, which facilitates a consistently high energy expenditure throughout the weight training period.

In a more recent study, Payne and Silvester (18) studied an exercise program that lasted from 18 to 36 minutes. The program consisted of 1 minute of jogging after each three stations of CWT (15 sec-per station). In addition to significantly improving strength, subjects improved aerobic capacity by 15 to 17 percent. Circuit weight training with intermittent jogging can have a significant effect on aerobic capacity.

Recent research shows that circuit weight training can improve one's aerobic capacity 5 to 15 percent.

Individuals who want dramatic improvement in aerobic power should undoubtedly go on aerobic conditioning programs. However, those wanting some aerobic fitness combined with improved strength may find circuit weight training to be a very effective program.

WEIGHT TRAINING AND WEIGHT CONTROL

Is aerobic exercise the only exercise we should use in considering a weight control program? Probably not. One important consideration when considering fat loss is that fat is burned in muscle tissue. Muscular people can burn more fat than those with less muscle. Another consideration in exercise and weight control is the concept of burning higher than basal-metabolic rate (bmr) amounts of fat during the post-exercise recovery period of heightened metabolic activity (discussed further below). An average individual burns approximately 100 calories while jogging or walking one mile. A 134 pound person would burn approximately 100 calories, and a 170 pound person would burn about 132 calories (1). Considering that there are 3600 calories in one pound of fat, it takes a considerable effort to lose one fat pound.

There is some evidence, albeit controversial evidence, that physical exercise, in addition to its direct caloric cost, also increases energy expenditure during the nonexercise recovery period. There is considerable uncertainty as to the degree and duration of the increase in metabolic rate after an exercise session. Some investigators have reported a rapid decline of the postexercise metabolic rate to basal levels (4, 10), whereas others have found an elevated metabolic rate 24 to 48 hours after exercise (3, 8).

ANAEROBIC EXERCISE AND WEIGHT CONTROL

Anaerobic exercise can be defined as exercise that uses oxygen at a rate faster than the body can supply it through respiratory processes. Thus, when we engage in anaerobic exercise we enter a state of oxygen debt. It is impossible for us to work anaerobically for more than about 45 seconds. Anaerobic exercise requires the expenditure of large amounts of energy in very short time periods. Lifting heavy weights, sprinting, and jumping are examples of such exercise.

If our basal metabolic rates are elevated for some time after aerobic exercise during which time we burn an increased number of fat calories (3, 8), it is logical to assume that the same condition must result from other types of exercise. The elevated metabolic rate after anaerobic exercise (weight training, basketball, racquetball, football, etc.) must also increase fat metabolism. Therefore such activity can be helpful in a weight control role.

Strength training can and does help a person control body fat. Consider for a moment individuals who engage in primarily anaerobic types of exercise: sprinters, weightlifters (consider all weight classes, not just the heavyweights), bodybuilders (even when not cutting up for a contest), and any other athlete in a basically nonaerobic activity. They usually have low levels of body fat. They may not appear as emaciated as elite distance runners—they do have reasonable body mass, but they usually have very low levels of body fat. Their condition undoubtedly results partly from heredity, partly from diet, and partly because *much of the time during most, primarily anaerobic, activities is spent at more moderate work rates when aerobic energy systems are functioning,* e.g., walking or jogging in basketball, standing between points in volleyball, walking to the baseline to serve in tennis, sitting or standing between sets in weight training.

Remember these important points about exercise:

1. Try to make the exercise vigorous. Build up a sweat and keep it going for most of the workout.

2. Find one or more vigorous activities you *enjoy,* jogging, tennis, racquetball, swimming, cycling, squash, badminton, cross-country skiing, weight training, basketball, hockey, soccer, aerobics, even walking, if done vigorously enough, will be be useful in your exercise program. The likelihood that you will continue with an exercise program increases dramatically if you enjoy it. (We all like the *results* of an exercise program. We feel good when the session is over, but sometimes we don't have the greatest love for the exercise program while it is in progress.)

3. When some fun activity is not readily available for fitness and you need a workout, discipline yourself to exercise anyway. Go jogging or walking, or run/walk the stairs, do calisthenics. You need it, you will feel better after doing it, and your life will be more enjoyable and productive.

FLEXIBILITY

At the 1972 Olympic Games, where I competed, a study was done that compared the flexibility of athletes in various events. The most flexible group were, predictably, the gymnasts. However, the Olympic weightlifters were second. I mention this only to further dispel the long-held concept that weight training (lifting) is associated with lack of flexibility. Weight training, if done properly, should improve flexibility!

Moving a resistance through a complete range of motion will challenge the flexibility of a joint both in full extension and full flexion. However, when weight training, there is a great temptation to cut short movements because we are generally stronger in the mid ranges than at the extremes of a range of motion. Do not give in to this temptation! Doing so for long enough can reduce the flexibility (range of motion) of a joint. Be conscientious about lifting a weight that is light enough that you can move it through the entire range of motion. Always use full range motion when weight training.

It is a good idea to make certain that muscles, tendons, and ligaments are warmed up before doing sets with 70 to 90 percent of 1RM. The best warmup is a set with relatively light weight (40 to 50 percent of the 1RM).

The best time to stretch is immediately after you have completed weight training or another exercise program. Your body is warmed up and should respond well to flexibility work. Doing flexibility movements while in a hot tub or a sauna is also considered advantageous because of the warmth associated with these environments. However, you can stretch anytime you choose. A good time to stretch might be when watching a TV program, or when talking to a friend who understands the importance of good physical fitness.

How to Improve Flexibility

Stretching is easy, but there are some things you should know before you begin. First, it is wise to stretch only to the point of *mild tension* on the muscles. I suppose some people could misinterpret "mild tension" and actually pull a muscle by stretching too intensely. Generally, you should not stretch to the point of pain. There is difference between tension and pain. If you choose to go into the pain zone occasionally, be certain that it is only mild pain. In most cases when you feel pain you have activated the stretch reflex (defined below), and the muscles you are trying to stretch are being stimulated with nervous impulses, causing them to contract. This condition is obviously counterproductive to improving flexibility and is potentially damaging to muscles, tendons, and ligaments.

The Stretch Reflex. Within muscle there are several proprioceptive structures known as muscle spindles. When a muscle is stretched beyond a certain normal level the muscle spindle fires, sending an impulse to the spinal cord where it is transferred to a motor neuron and sent back to the muscle as a signal to the muscle to contract. The stretch reflex is considered to be primarily a mechanism to protect the muscle from overstretch and possible injury. When stretching to maintain or improve flexibility we want to avoid activating this reflex.

How often should you stretch? A good answer is that you should consider stretching as often as is practical. Once per day is a worthwhile objective. However, twice per day is better, particularly if you are trying to improve flexibility. As we age we tend to lose flexibility; therefore, stretching frequency should be increased for us to remain supple.

Remember these important concepts about flexibility work:

1. Regularity is paramount. You must be consistent for a considerable period of time to expect significant improvement in flexibility.
2. Learning to relax the muscles while stretching is a demanding skill. You need to learn this before your flexibility increases. Generally this involves feeling the point of mild tension which, if held for 15 to 20 seconds, allows you to relax the muscle and stretch a little bit more and still feel comfortable. Learning your own comfortable limits and knowing your body is important.
3. Don't bounce while stretching. Bouncing has the effect of activating the stretch reflex.
4. As you go through the various stretches you will start to develop a feeling of just how you get the most out of the flexibility movements. It is important that you are aware of proper body alignment and positions. Each change results in a slightly different application of the stretching forces. You are the creator; be sensitive as you experiment with different feelings.

The following flexibility movements can help you stretch most of the major areas of the body:

1. Elbow above head, pulled behind by opposite hand (latissimus dorsi-tricep) (See Figure 3–4).
2. Arm ventrally across upper chest, pulled by opposite arm (latissimus dorsi-tricep) (See Figure 3–5).

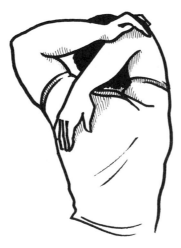

Figure 3–4
Latissimus dorsi-tricep stretch

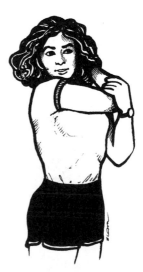

Figure 3–5
Latissimus dorsi-tricep stretch

Figure 3–6
Latissimus dorsi-
tricep strech

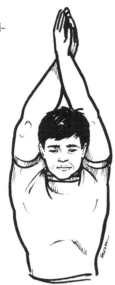

Figure 3–7
Anterior-superior
deltoid, pec
major, and
bicep stretch

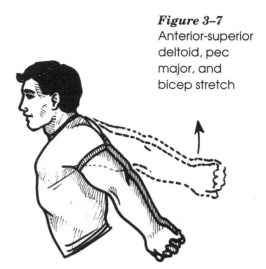

3. Arms above head, hands clasped in inverted grip (latissimus dorsi-tricep) (See Figure 3–6).
4. Arms behind back, raised up (anterior- superior deltoid, pec major, biceps) (See Figure 3–7).
5. Side bends (sides of upper body) (See Figure 3–8).
6. Adductor stretch—feet spread, bend down on one knee and stretch the inside of the opposite leg (adductors) (See Figure 3–9).

Figure 3–8
Side Bends

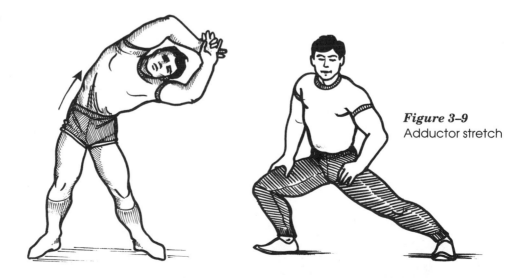

Figure 3–9
Adductor stretch

Figure 3–10
Adductor stretch

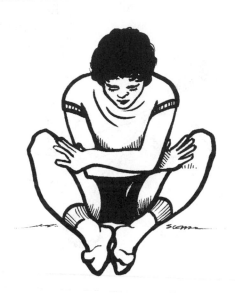

Figure 3–11
Stretch for
lateral hip,
sides–lats,
deltoid, and
tricep

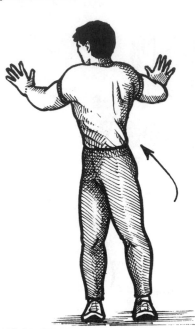

7.   Sitting feet together, apply downward pressure gently on knees
     (See Figure 3–10).
8.   Hip twist—feet shoulder-width apart facing away from wall. Turn
     your upper body and put your hands on the wall. Head and
     shoulders face the wall, but feet point directly away from the wall
     (lateral hip, sides-lats, deltoid and triceps) (See Figure 3–11).
9.   Spinal twist (See Figure 3–12).

Figure 3–12
Spinal Twist

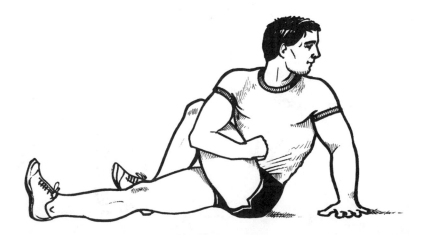

Figure 3-13
Back, buttocks,
and hamstring
stretch

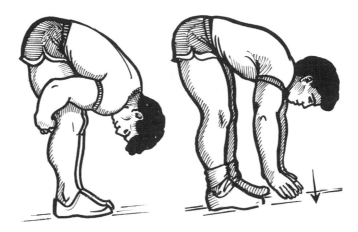

10. Back, buttocks, and hamstring stretch—bend forward, touch hands on toes or floor, then wrap arms around legs about knee level; pull with arms to stretch the back (See Figure 3–13).
11. Sitting cross legged, leaning forward, stretching back and buttocks (See Figure 3–14).
12. Sitting, legs forward, stretch the hamstrings (See Figure 3–15).
13. Quadriceps stretch—lift foot up behind your leg, grasp it in the hand and pull the heel up against the buttocks (See Figure 3–16).

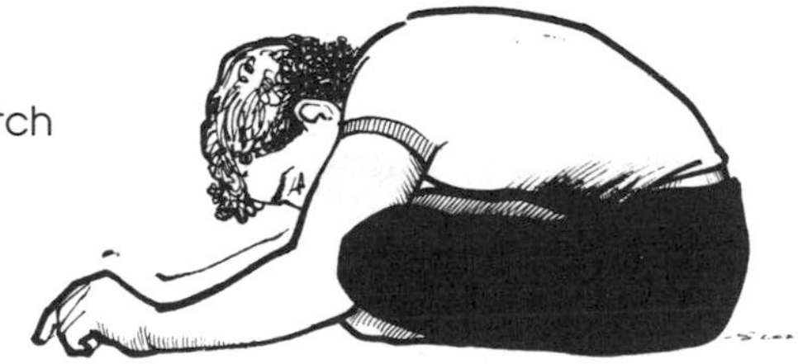

Figure 3-14
Back and
buttocks stretch

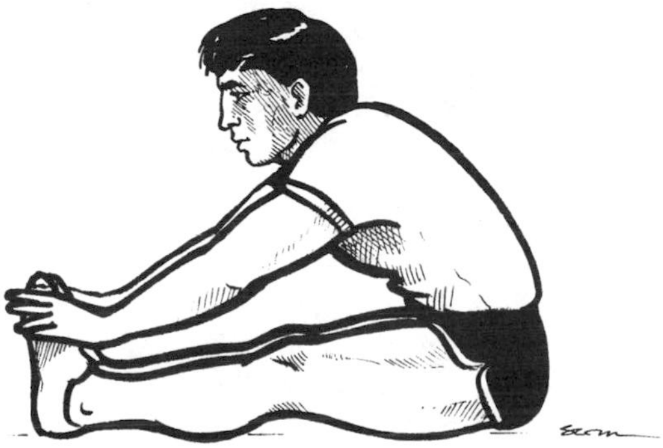

Figure 3-15
Hamstring
stretch

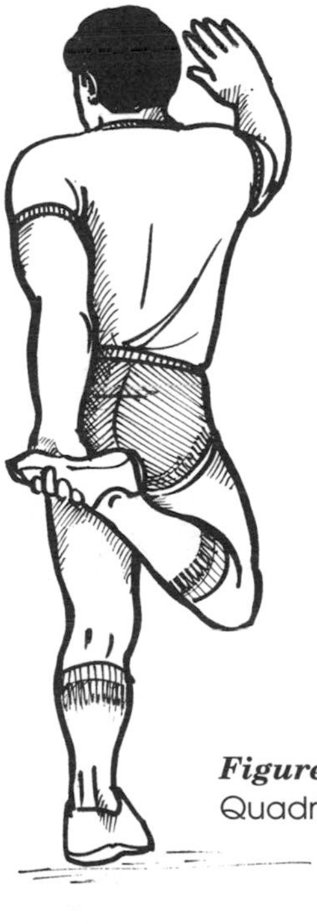

Figure 3-16
Quadricep stretch

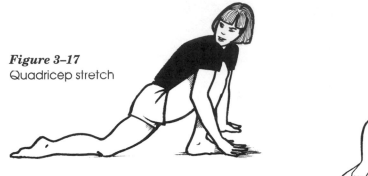

Figure 3–17
Quadricep stretch

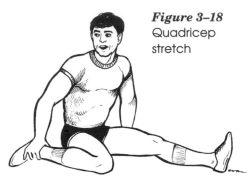

Figure 3–18
Quadricep
stretch

14. One leg back, knee down (ventrally), other leg with knee against chest (quadricep stretch for the rear leg) (See Figure 3–17).
15. Hurdle position, lean back and stretch the quadriceps, as opposed to the hamstrings (rear leg) (See Figure 3–18).
16. Gastrocnemius and soleus stretch—stand three or four feet away from a wall. Lean against the wall, supporting your body with your hands. Move your feet as far back away from the wall as possible while keeping the heels down (See Figure 3–19).
17. Sitting with one leg forward, and toes up, pull toes back gently with a towel (See Figure 3–20).

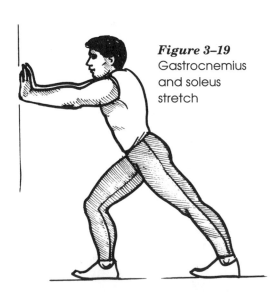

Figure 3–19
Gastrocnemius
and soleus
stretch

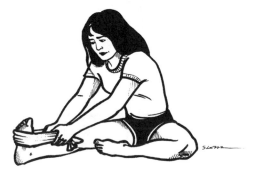

Figure 3–20
Toe stretch

POSITIVE ADDICTION TO EXERCISE

Many activities in life have the potential to become somewhat captivating to human beings. Art, literature, theater, music, dance, and of course all sports qualify as candidates for our special attention. It is not a long step from being captivated by an activity to becoming compulsively involved in it. Becoming psychologically or physiologically compelled to behave in a particular way is often referred to as being addicted.

You may have heard the phrase *positive addiction* used to describe someone who is so taken with a particular physical activity (usually jogging) that he or she does it compulsively. If such people go a day or two without working out they feel quite uncomfortable. If the condition is not extreme it may be very beneficial in helping a person keep physically fit. As with all compulsive behavior, however, if we lose control the results are usually quite detrimental. Unfortunately, some individuals have lost jobs, friends, and in some cases physical well-being by spending many hours each day in compulsive exercise and sport sessions.

Exercise to maintain good health should not require more than one hour per day. On the other hand, the workout requirements to be a competitive athlete can be as high as four to five hours per day. Physical fitness and athletic training are uniquely different endeavors.

WEIGHT CONTROL AND NUTRITION

The present generally accepted guideline for a proper mix of calories in our diets is carbohydrates 48 percent, simple sugars (refined carbohydrates) 10 percent, fats 30 percent, and protein 12 percent (14, 20). It is important to understand that when we discuss these proportions, we are discussing the caloric content of the foods, not the weight of foods or their volume. A baked potato with a precooked weight of eight ounces has about 132 calories of carbohydrate, 16 calories of protein, and no fat (not considering the skin). If you add one pat of butter (one fifth of an ounce), you add 36 calories of fat. This changes the caloric ratio of the potato from zero percent fat to 19 percent. Two pats of butter put the ratio up to 32 percent fat. If you then add a tablespoon of sour cream, the ratio goes to 39 percent fat. In this case, 99 of 247 calories are fat. Adding cheese increases the percentage of fat even more. Many calories are packed into small volumes of fat. The same is generally true of simple sugar.

When we get hungry we need volume as well as calories. If our diets contain high fat, simple sugar, or both, we can consume many calories before we get a feeling of being full. Many people frequently eat in such a manner. One of the keys to good nutrition is to assure that our diets contain large amounts of complex carbohydrates: vegetables, fruits, and breads.

When we get hungry we need volume as well as calories. If our diets contain high fat and/or simple sugar, we can consume huge numbers of calories before we get a feeling of being full.

The way foods high in fats and sugars are prepared usually makes them *taste very good*. As a result, most of us enjoy eating such foods. However, if we are to live healthfully, we need to resist that desire. Such avoidance becomes a matter of lifelong self-control. How are we as a population doing in our efforts to resist unhealthy eating? Not as well as we might.

It has been reported for some years now that the average American diet contains too much fat. The average American diet contains around 40 percent fat. The American Dietetic Association and the American Medical Association recommend no more than 30 percent fat and the American Heart Association suggests not more than 25 percent fat. Nathan Pritikin, a researcher in nutrition, recommends a very low 10 to 15 percent fat.

The problem is not entirely with the fast-food restaurants, the ice cream vendors, or the consumer. Each of these elements, plus other forces in our society, share some of the blame for our lack of nutritional understanding and control.

Most Americans are not taught how to prepare nutritionally well-balanced meals. How many of us have sat through exciting and memorable classes in the nutritional content of various foods? How many have studied how to prepare foods in delicious, nutritious, exciting, and quick ways? Anyone? How many of us have taken the time to read and study at least one good nutrition book? Though this subject is important, most of us don't give it a very high priority.

DETERMINING RECOMMENDED BODY WEIGHT AND BODY COMPOSITION

Most of us have seen charts that suggest ranges of body weight for various heights. These charts give us guidelines, but they are not very accurate. Body weight in relation to height is important, but it is more important to know the percentage of our total weight that is fat. It is not unusual to meet the criteria on the height weight charts but still have considerably more fat than is desirable (1).

The amount of body fat that enables a particular individual to enjoy optimal health and fitness is not something that can be precisely deter-

Table 3-1 General Guidelines of Fat Levels
for Males and Females (percentages)

	Males	Females
Too little fat	0-4	0-12
Appropriate fat	5-15	13-23
Somewhat overfat	16-24	24-32
Obese	24+	33+

mined. Ranges have been established as general guidelines (See Table 3-1), but determining *precisely* what level of fat a person should have is currently beyond our predictive ability. (Note that women are genetically endowed with fat levels 7 to 8 percent higher than men.)

Once we know what a desirable percentage of body fat is we often want to know our body composition. Researchers have found different techniques for estimating body-fat levels. The most precise method of determining body composition is hydrostatic or underwater weighing. This technique is based on the concept that fat floats and lean body mass does not. Lean body weight determined in underwater weighing compared to total weight results in a pretty accurate fat percentage. This method requires expensive equipment, immersion in water, and considerable time.

By *measuring skinfold thicknesses* at various sites and carefully correlating these measures with hydrostatic weighing, physiologists have developed relatively accurate charts for estimating body-fat levels. This is a simple technique. The skinfold calipers necessary for this procedure are available at the departments of exercise science or physical education at most colleges and universities. Other techniques for estimating body composition include bioelectrical impedance and using ultrasonic sound waves.

PROTEIN

Do athletes or others who exercise frequently require more protein than a "normal diet" provides?

The recommended dietary allowance (RDA) for protein is 0.8 grams of protein per kilogram of body weight per day. Grandjean and his coresearchers suggested that 0.8 grams may not be adequate for the active individual (11). Dohm reviewed and summarized various studies that considered the adequacy of the protein RDA for athletes. He recommended that athletes consume 1.0 to 1.5 grams of protein per kilogram of body weight (9). His recommendation does exceed the RDA, but the average self-selected American diet contains 15 percent protein (about 2.0 g of protein per kg per day). Most of us, including the hard-working athlete, are exceeding our protein requirements. Protein powders, pills, and drinks that are consumed in addition to the normal diet profit the manufacturer and provide no apparent physiological benefit to the consumer.

Free amino acids, which have become popular in the past few years as a source of nutrients more easily available to the body than intact proteins, are also suspect as a nutritional advantage. For more than 99 percent of Americans dietary amino acids are supplied as proteins. Since the body is very efficient at breaking down the proteins and absorbing the resultant amino acids (16), there is no reason to suggest that free amino acids offer any advantage over amino acids that result from the digestion of proteins.

SLEEP AND REST

Fitness and rest are inseparable. To develop a high level of physical fitness a person must either have or develop good rest habits. Sleep is considered the most important component of rest. Some time ago I was asked by a student who had been training for about eight weeks, "When will I start needing less sleep?" I responded that nothing I have read or experienced suggests that improved fitness would reduce required amounts of sleep or rest.

> To develop high levels of physical fitness a person must either have or develop good rest habits.

My own experience suggests that heavy athletic training requires most athletes to *increase* their rest time. Such training is certainly more demanding than a fitness routine, but even a fitness workout may cause a person to sleep longer or take a nap sometime during the day, particularly when a person begins such a program. We often hear testimonials that fitness programs help individuals get better quality sleep. Most people believe that the body is more relaxed after a day that includes a reasonably vigorous workout. *Very few people would disagree that consistent exercise programs are associated with quality sleep habits.* However, working out late in the evening can elevate your metabolic rate and make it difficult to wind down. Exercise sessions that are completed 2 or more hours before bedtime are normally not a problem.

Naps are great when needed. To have the opportunity to lie down for a few minutes when we strongly feel the need is a great blessing. These brief rest breaks generally should not last for more than 20 to 30 minutes. Napping for longer periods often results in feeling groggy and slowed down as opposed to refreshed and energized.

WEIGHT TRAINING AND STRESS MANAGEMENT

Weight training can help anyone feel less stressed after a workout than they were before the exercise session. This is accomplished primarily in two ways. First, focusing for a period of time on the workout routine takes your thoughts off the problems of the day. Second, after completing a good exercise routine and a good shower, you feel relaxed and calmer than at most other times. This break from the major stressors in life can reduce their intensity and even offer opportunities for a new and fresh view of the problem once you get back to work. Most physically demanding exercise routines or sports have this same potential.

REFERENCES

1. Allsen, P. E., J. M. Harrison, and B. Vance. 1976. *Fitness for Life: An Individualized Approach.* Dubuque, Iowa: Wm. C. Brown.
2. American College of Sports Medicine. 1978. vii–x.
3. Bielinski, R., Y. Schutz, and E. Jequer. 1985. Energy metabolism during the postexercise recovery in man. *American Journal of Clinical Nutrition* 42: 69–82.
4. Brehm, B.A., and B. Gutin, 1986. Recovery energy expenditure for steady state exercise in runners and nonexercisers. *Medicine and Science in Sports and Exercise* 18: 205–210.
5. Clarke, H. H., ed. 1971. The totality of man. *Physical Fitness Research Digest* Series 1, no. 2.
6. Cooper, K. 1977. *The Aerobics Way.* New York: M. Evans Co.
7. Cureton, T. K. 1973. *The Physiological Effects of Exercise Programs on Adults.* Springfield, Ill.: Charles C. Thomas.
8. deVries, H. A., and D. E. Gray, 1963. Aftereffects of exercise on resting metabolic rate. *Research Quarterly* 34: 314–321.
9. Dohm, G. L. 1984. Protein nutrition for the athlete. In A. Hecker (ed.), *Nutritional Aspects of Exercise: Clinical Sports Medicine.* Philadelphia: Saunders.
10. Friedman-Akabas, S., E. Colt, H. R. Kissleff, and F. X. Pi-Sunyer. 1985. Lack of sustained increase in VO2 following exercise in fit and unfit subjects. *American Journal of Clinical Nutrition* 41: 545–549.
11. Grandjean, A. C., L. M. Hursh, et al., 1981. Nutrition knowledge and practices of college athletes. *Medicine and Science in Sports and Exercise* 13: 82.
12. Gettman, L. R., and M. L. Pollock. 1981. Circuit weight training: A critical review of its physiological benefits. *The Physician and Sports Medicine.* 9 (1): 44–60.

13. Hempel, L. S., and C. L. Wells. 1985. Cardiorespiratory cost of Nautilus express circuit. *The Physician and Sports Medicine* 13: 4.

14. Hui, Y. H. 1985. *Principles and Issues in Nutrition.* Boston: Jones and Bartlett.

15. Karvonen, M., K. Kentala, and O. Mustala. 1957. The effects of training on heart rate: A longitudinal study. *Annales Medicinal Experimentales Biologial Fennial (Finnish Journal of Experimental Medicine)* 35: 305–315.

16. Kasperek, G. J. 1988. Amino acid metabolism. *NSCA Journal* 10: 6.

17. Kraus, H., and W. Raab. 1961. *Hypokinetic Disease.* Springfield Ill.: Charles C. Thomas.

18. Payne, C., and L. J. Silvester. 1989. The effectiveness of a circuit weight training program with intermittent running on strength, cardiorespiratory endurance, and body composition. Masters thesis, Brigham Young University, Provo, Utah.

19. Stone, M. H., and H. O'Bryant. 1987. *Weight Training: A Scientific Approach.* Minneapolis: Bellweather Press.

20. U.S. Senate Select Committee on Nutrition and Human Needs. 1977. Dietary goals for the United States.

CHAPTER FOUR

Strength Fitness and Bodybuilding (Body Sculpting)

STRENGTH FITNESS WEIGHT TRAINING

A fifty-year-old grandmother of four came to my office to discuss weight training. She was tall and rather lean and her blonde hair was streaked with grey. The slight curvature in her upper spine suggested the beginning of osteoporosis. She seemed the perfect candidate for such a problem: obvious Scandinavian lineage, thin features, and very close to menopause. She was nervous. It had taken some courage to decide to discuss some ideas with a "professional." She said her husband, a friend of mine, had suggested that she come to see me. After some time she decided to do what he had recommended.

Her major concern was that she not lose any more strength. She had four grandchildren, three of whom lived near her. She loved being with them but found it difficult to play with them and particularly to lift them. She wondered if some weight training would help her with that and just help her feel a little better in general. I asked her a few questions about her lifestyle. Had she ever been physically active? Had she played on some sports team in school or in some recreational league? Her answers to these questions were generally negative. She had never been on a sports team when she was younger; very few girls were when she was in high school and college. She had made sporadic attempts to get and stay fit, but the pressures of raising a family, holding part time jobs, and then helping her children and grandchildren had preempted the time she might have spent in a consistent exercise program.

Her story is not uncommon. Most women of her generation would probably tell one similar to it. Exercise and fitness were not high priorities. We in the fitness business think things are better in the 1990s.

She and I talked about time to exercise, committment to a program and someone to workout with—an important help when starting a new activity. We decided that she would enroll in an evening weight training class. I suggested that if she would be consistent for three months she would feel much better and would probably be converted to the good feelings associated with regular exercise for the rest of her life. As the semester progressed I counseled her about an aerobic program. She decided to start riding an exercycle in the weight room for 20 minutes after each class (three times per week).

Three months later she did feel better, although the changes were not as dramatic as I had hoped. She had gained some strength, but her heredity, age, and attitude had not been the best for producing the greatest possible change. It would to take longer for her to change than I had expected. However, she had been consistent. She had kept her end of the bargain. She had tried, and the results were obvious. Her strength had improved but she had not learned to enjoy exercise. She had to more or less force herself to weight train; it was not an activity she looked forward to excitedly.

I see her husband occasionally at my work. We sometimes discuss her attention to weight training and general fitness. Shortly after the class they purchased an exercycle and a home gym (multistation weightlifting machine), and she has been consistent in working on and improving her fitness ever since.

This story is about someone who is more or less middle of the road in terms of the success of the program. Others with whom I have worked have been highly successful and one person with whom I have counselled has given up weight training entirely. This woman sticks with her program because she realizes that doing so is important to her well-being. She has the self-discipline to do what needs doing, an admirable characteristic for anyone.

There are other stories, many others. One young man was thin and intelligent, but very weak. He was listless when I met him. A few months later, with a healthy diet, weight training, other fitness activities, and proper rest he had a bright, twinkling eye, and a happy countenance. He felt great! An overweight girl lost 30 pounds in one semester, improved her strength by about 20 percent, and was still with the program three years later.

Each of these people engaged in what I refer to as *strength fitness exercise*. Strength fitness is for all ages (after about age eight), shapes, and sizes. Strength fitness exercise is the weight training approach for the masses. This is the program for the busy businessman who can spend 30 minutes two to three times per week, and for the high school or college student who wants to remain firm and "toned." It is also the program for the homemaker and her neighbor, the hairdresser. It is the best approach to maintaining a reasonable strength level for those millions employed in American industry and the military services. It includes the type of training that young boys or girls might engage in as they *begin* strength training to improve their athletic potential. For 95 to 99 percent of the population in the United States strength fitness exercise is the most logical approach to getting and keeping the body fit and strong.

Strength fitness exercise is the best weight training approach for the majority of people.

What are the specifics of a strength fitness program? There is no single weight training program for strength fitness. Rather, there are many weight training routines that a person might design that would fall into the strength fitness category. The following criteria identify a strength fitness weight training routine.

1. The resistance levels (amount of weight used) or intensity level in this type of program is purposely *moderate*. This is not to say that a strength fitness workout is not vigorous exercise—when done properly, it is—but the resistance levels used generally do not exceed 85 percent of the 1RM and are seldom that high.
2. Each set requires from 6 to 15 or possibly 20 (for some muscle groups) repetitions.
3. Each set is carried to a point either at or very near momentary muscular failure.
4. Workouts generally do not last more than 30 to 45 minutes.
5. Exercises in the routine affect all the major muscles of the body.
6. The frequency of workout could be six or seven times per week, but three times is quite adequate.

People involved in this type of workout are not interested in maximizing strength, they are interested in maximizing *strength fitness*. They want good health and a fit body. They know that it does not require long, arduous hours of effort to achieve or to maintain quite satisfactory levels of fitness. They know one of the great secrets of overall well-being: they need to spend some time and effort working on all of the important areas of life but not spend inordinate amounts of time maximizing any one aspect, fitness included. Various exercises and set-repetition combinations might be used that would result in essentially the same strength fitness level. Two examples are as follows:

Strength Fitness Program 1

Exercise	# sets	#reps
Shoulder shrugs	3	8
Upright rows	3	8
Dumbbell curls	3	8
Tricep pressdown	3	8
Supine flies	3	8
Seated cable rows	3	8
Abdominal curls	2	25
Hip extension	3	10
Hip flexion	3	10
Leg extension	3	8
Leg curl	3	8
Heel raises	3	20

Strength Fitness Program 2

Exercise	# sets	#reps
Side lat. raise	2	12
Bent over row	2	12
Curl machine curl	2	12
O/h tricep press	2	12
Bench press	2	12
Lat. pulldown	2	12
Crunch situps	2	30
Leg extension	2	12
Leg curl	2	12
Hip extension	2	12
Hip flexion	2	12
Toe presses	2	20

Notice there are three sets in the first program and only two in the second. Also notice that the repetitions are fewer in the three-set program. The three-set program requires more work than does the two-set routine but, as *strength fitness weight training programs,* both are quite appropriate. When writing a weight training program in the above manner (sets followed by a number of repetitions) it is assumed that the exerciser is using an amount of resistance (weight) that causes the last repetition of the set to be at, or very close to, momentary muscular failure.

Momentary Muscular Failure

The phenomenon of momentary muscular failure is momentary failure of the energy supplying systems of the body. This condition in weight training is brought on by brief unrelenting exercise of a muscle group. It has been said that *the most important repetition in a set is the last one.* This idea is based on the premise that the last repetition is the most painful one and therefore the one that sends the strongest signal(s) to the body to adapt (become stronger, more fit/or toned). The last repetition may indeed result in the strongest message being sent to those receptors responsible for change; there is no research corroborating or negating such a thesis. However, since all the preceding repetitions are necessary to finally arrive at that last one, it is obvious that all are of equal importance. One simply cannot occur without the other.

WEIGHT TRAINING AT OR CLOSE TO FATIGUE LEVELS

Let us carefully consider a concept closely related to the one just discussed. If the last repetition is the most important, or possibly the last two or three during which the pain is the most intense, why rest and recover before doing the next set? Why not just take a very brief rest so that you can only do two or three repetitions in the next set, with a weight that you could lift at least eight repetitions in a recovered state. A person using this system would purposely try to keep exercising in a rather fatigued state. Once again, there is no research on this possible exercise routine. It seems unlikely that there ever will be. Such a routine would be extremely painful to endure and mentally painful to contemplate. Such a routine could not be engaged in for very long, even by the most highly motivated: the psychological and physical stress would simply become unbearable. Further, the systems of the body would not adapt and improve under such stress but would instead begin to deteriorate as they moved into what Selye described as the exhaustion stage of the General Adaptation Syndrome (3). (See Figure 2–8 on page 31.) Muscular fatigue should be experienced only very briefly at or near the end of each set.

> Working at or near fatigue levels is appropriate, but only when those fatigue levels are experienced briefly at or near the end of a set that began in a refreshed or reasonably recovered state.

BODYBUILDING AND BODY SCULPTING

Although bodybuilding and body sculpting have certain characteristics in common, they mean different things. *Bodybuilding* is the terminology that has been used since the time of Eugene Sandow (see Chapter One) to describe the activity of those who are interested in producing physiques of extreme musculature. *Body sculpting* is a term of relatively recent genesis, which is used liberally by the health spa industry to attract (primarily women) to their businesses. Body sculpting refers more to trimming, tightening, or toning the body than to building massive musculature. Bodybuilding implies the building of massive musculature and body symmetry, while body sculpting suggests building an attractive shapely physique without excessive muscularity. Certainly, bodybuilders sculpt their bodies, but their objective is quite unlike that of most fitness enthusiasts. Chapter One contains a brief introduction to bodybuilding and a brief history of the activity.

Below is a description of the workout of two young men who have become impassioned with bodybuilding. It is offered to help you understand the activity.

Two relatively muscular young men enter the weight room. Both are greeted briefly by others already there. They are in a university weight room that is well equipped with barbells, dumbbells, benches, mirrors, and various exercise machines. Four or five athletes are working out on the squat racks and two more are doing cleans. Most of the other twenty-plus people are engaged in strength fitness work. There is a different air about the two who have just entered the room. They immediately set to work.

Heel high (crunch) sit-ups first: three sets of 75 reps, and then three sets of 80, alternated with sets of leg raises, with no more than one minute between sets. They work very precisely, not bouncing, but working the muscle through each inch of the range. They make their muscles pump,

Figure 4–1
Bodybuilders
working
together doing
crunch sit-ups

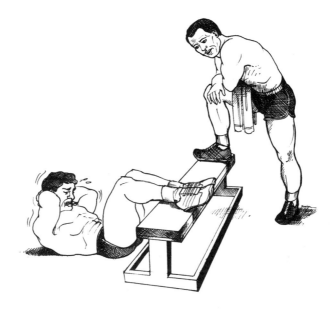

make them hurt, get the pump going. They follow sit-ups with rapid torso twists: they use a bar across the shoulders, sit on a bench, and spin back and forth to work the obliques and the lower back area. After four sets of twists, thirty intense minutes of work have passed, and they are ready to go on to a more enjoyable part of the workout, the arms.

Each man takes an E-Z curl bar, loads it to 100 pounds, does one set of 10, adds 10 pounds, does two sets of 9, adds 10 pounds, then does three sets of 8. Then they move to a dumbbell rack where each does a set of dumbbell curls alternating with sets of inner curls on the preacher board: five sets of each, between 8 and 12 reps in each set. Man, are those biceps pumped!

Triceps are next: triceps pressdown, five sets of 8, then a decline tricep press, one set of 10 followed by four sets of 8 at 10 pounds heavier weight. Five 10 rep sets of tricep pulley extensions using the universal machine round out the workout on the arms. The arms of the two men are pumped and bulging, particularly the triceps.

They work their legs next, starting with front squats: one set of 20 at 190, one set of 12 at 220, then three sets of 10 at 250. Lunges are next, five sets of 10, with 130, then they alternate leg extensions (12 reps/set) and leg curls (10 reps/set), four sets of each. Make it burn—develop those thighs!

After the thigh work, both men, sweating steadily, move to the universal gym leg press station. The weight is set at 280 pounds, and they begin doing toe presses: sets of 20 alternating from heels inverted to heels turned out to heels in a middle position. They go through eight sets.

Finished with the toe presses, they move to a platform where with one leg at a time they do heel raises while holding a 50 pound dumbbell in the hand on the same side as the working calf. Six sets later they replace the dumbbells, bid a few people farewell, and leave the room.

Their workout required about one hour and thirty minutes of intense, concentrated effort. They will return again the next day to concentrate on different body parts. However, the abdominal work will be similar: they work the abdominals every day. They are working a split routine, six days per week, same body parts every other day.

These two college students realize that two hours of work per day cuts into their study time, but they have been bitten by the bodybuilding bug, so they are giving it a go. They are training for a couple of local contests. Maybe they will make it, maybe they won't, but for now they are into bodybuilding. If one or both are successful in their initial competitive efforts, they will likely continue and seek greater challenges. If not (and most are not) the obsession will gradually wear off, and working with weights will assume a much less important place in their lives.

The workout described above is that of a reasonably fit bodybuilder. It is impressive to observe the work capacity of such individuals. A successful bodybuilder must have other characteristics in addition to a great capacity for work. *Probably the most important are relatively broad shoulders, narrow hips, and the ability to produce large muscle mass.* Only about 3 to 5 percent of the male population of the United States have these characteristics. If you were not blessed with them it is best that you enjoy your workouts but not aspire to competition in bodybuilding.

The objectives of a bodybuilder are to develop (1) maximum muscle size, (2) bodily symmetry (proportion), (3) definition, and (4) vascularity. To achieve these objectives all successful bodybuilders must be disciplined and very highly motivated.

Their workouts require stringent consistency and high pain tolerance, but their dietary control may be even more demanding. Six to eight weeks before important competitions, bodybuilders reduce fat and carbohydrate levels in their diets to almost zero. This practice ultimately removes most of the subcutaneous fat from the body, thereby thinning the skin and allowing the musculature to be displayed in the most advantageous manner.

MUSCULAR HYPERTROPHY

Bodybuilders give inclandestine expression to an innate male desire to be imposing or domineering simply by physical appearance. This is not to say that males don't desire to back up appearance with ability to perform; they do. Having a powerful appearance and being able to perform well in sport or physical combat is a very desirable combination of male traits.

Anyone who has been involved in strength training for thirty-five years, as I have, has observed that if males age fifteen through thirty persist in a strength training program hypertrophy results from any set-repetition combination where repetitions are kept at 15 or less. This same person has also developed the feeling that strength levels are best improved by working in the range of 3 to 6 reps, with an occasional foray into 1-rep maxes.

This person would also be aware that bodybuilders usually do more repetitions (8–12), with necessarily lighter percentages of their maximum lift levels, than the 3 to 6 repetition work characteristic of athletes or competitive lifters.

Enter L. Matveyev and, subsequently, John Garhammer, Michael Stone, and others proposing the periodization model of strength training (2, 5). The periodization model includes time in a training cycle devoted to work at essentially all repetition levels, from a high of 8 to 12 to a low of 1 to 3. The basis for including the high repetition work lies in the concept that there is a relationship between the strength of a muscle and the size of a muscle. The current belief is that once a muscle has reached a hypothetical maximum strength level, strength can only be improved by (1) increasing the number of muscle fibers (hyperplasia) or (2) increasing the size of the muscle fibers already present. Either condition would increase total muscle mass. High repetition work (8–12 reps) has been shown to maximize hypertrophy (1). Somewhat curiously, the workout routine which maximizes hypertrophy does not maximize strength. Therefore, those wishing to maximize strength need to engage in a periodized regimen. Conversely, bodybuilders would probably not drop below the 8RM level in their workouts.

An enlightening research study by Kraemer and Fleck (1) showed that when participants did three to five sets of their 10RM with only 1 minute rest between sets, blood testosterone levels were elevated. When subjects were allowed 3 or more minutes of rest between sets, blood testosterone levels dropped significantly. The exact relationship between muscle mass and testosterone levels is not known, but it is assumed that high levels of testosterone facilitate the building of muscle mass in humans.

ANABOLIC STEROIDS IN BODYBUILDING

Anabolic steroids are synthetic derivatives of the male hormone testosterone. Use of the drug causes a positive nitrogen balance in the cell, which can facilitate the addition of muscle mass. The use of anabolic steroids is rampant among bodybuilders, as it is among many athletes in strength-power events. Aspiring bodybuilders must make a decision whether or not to use these much abused drugs. Unfortunately, most bodybuilders think a person cannot be successful without their use. See Chapter Two for a more thorough discussion of anabolic steroids.

BASIC BODYBUILDING CONCEPTS

1. All of the major muscle groups should be developed for symmetry, proportion, size, and definition.
2. Each repetition should be performed observing strict technique.
3. The "pump" is the desired goal. Do what is necessary to get a good pump. Though there is no scientific definition of the pump a bodybuilder achieves, it seems to be a combination of engorging a muscle with blood and partial muscular tetany. When a muscle is pumped, it feels tight and is definitely larger than when it is in a relaxed state. The pump, essential for making physiological progress, is very positive mental feedback to the bodybuilder.

4. A serious bodybuilder must see his or her progress. Goals, records of progress, and measurements are very important.

5. Train for bulk for an appropriate period of time. (This time is different for different individuals.) Then go on a workout for definition and carefully control your diet six to eight weeks prior to a contest. The amount of weight you will lose when cutting up, as definition training is called, may vary from 10 to 20 pounds. Bodybuilders would hope this weight loss would be entirely body fat.

6. Posing is an art form that successful bodybuilders must master. A bodybuilder must have a posing repertoire that displays his or her body in the most advantageous way. The posing routine, which should last about 15 minutes, should be smooth, fluid, and relaxed with equal time for each pose. Developing a good posing routine requires considerable time and help from someone knowledgable in posing technique.

This, then, has been a brief description of some of the serious bodybuilders' activities and concerns. For those who are gifted, bodybuilding can be an intriguing and worthwhile experience. For those of us who are not so gifted, it is probably best that our conditioning be less intense and directed at keeping our bellies flat and our limbs firm.

DEVELOPING A NICE-LOOKING PHYSIQUE

What does it take to develop a nice-looking physique? The serious bodybuilder may spend from 3 to 6 hours per day exercising in a rigorously disciplined way, concentrating on various areas of the physique. Someone who is highly motivated to change appearance may devote those amounts of time, but the majority of us will not. An hour per day devoted to a well-designed workout routine will significantly affect most people's appearance within about three months. After one year of consistent workouts, the improvements should be quite obvious and pleasing. Our heredity, of course, significantly affects our appearance. Attempting to change one's inherited appearance is possible, but only within certain reasonable limits (see the discussion on body types that follows). Any attempt to change one's appearance requires stringent workouts, careful attention to diet, and adequate rest. Eating the right foods can help us put on lean body mass if we are too thin and lose adipose tissue if we need to do so.

An hour per day devoted to a well-designed workout *routine* will have a significant effect on the appearance of most people within about three months.

The workout exercises for developing a nice physique are no different than those for improving fitness. (See Chapter Four for weight training routines that can produce such effects).

BODY TYPES AND A NICE-LOOKING PHYSIQUE

Understanding different body types and how they generally respond to attempts to change them helps as you undertake such a project. It is obvious that we have different appearances. Body typing began in order to categorize these appearances and to assess their effects on our lives.

The individual most recognized for his work in this area is William H. Sheldon (4). During the blastula stage of embryonic development, a fertilized human ovum has three identifiable layers. The ectoderm, or outer layer, is the portion from which the skin, hair, nails, and other outer structures of the body arise. The mesoderm is the middle portion, from which our muscle, nerves, and bone generally develop. And the inner layer, or endoderm, is that portion from which the internal organs of the body originate. To Sheldon, bodies can be typed by assessing the contributions to the total body makeup of the various layers that are observable during the blastula stage. (See Figure 4–2.) Tall, thin individuals are more predominantly covering (skin); thus they are referred to as *ectomorphs*. The heavily muscled, husky person has a preponderance of muscle and bone; therefore they are designated *mesomorphs*. And heavy-set people with protruding

Figure 4–2
William
Sheldon's body
types

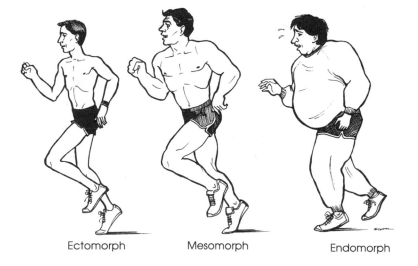

Ectomorph   Mesomorph   Endomorph

abdomens have a preponderance of internal mass (organs); therefore they are referred to as *endomorphs.*

Ectomorphs usually want to add some muscle to their frames. With concentrated effort, arduous work, and careful attention to diet they can make some improvement in muscularity. Mesomorphic men are generally pleased with their builds, while women in this category sometimes want to trim their legs and hips. Though a formidable task, it can be done with carefully planned exercise routines and perserverance. Endomorphs usually want to lose fat and put on muscle. This is also difficult but possible, with consistent work and self-discipline.

Changing one's physical appearance is not easy. It requires motivation that results in consistent exercise and disciplined eating habits. The actual requirements to produce changes in appearance differ from one person to another depending on our heredity, beginning fitness levels, lifestyle, and level of motivation. Should you decide to make some changes, it is a good idea to find out specifically where you are now (body measurements, including weight and perhaps strength levels) and then set some specific goals. It is also helps to have some model in mind that you aspire to look like. Who is your model?

Heredity largely determines what we look like. We can, through intense exercise and extreme self-discipline, change our muscular appearance and our posture when we are in our youth, but without consistent effort and attention these changes may not be evident as we age.

Everyone would like to have what he or she considers a nice-looking physique—or at least a body that does not cause him or her embarassment. But for most people there is a time in life when we want more from our bodies than just self-satisfaction. We want our physiques to help us in attracting and holding the attention of the opposite sex. This is not to suggest that anyone spend hours of time each day exercising and grooming and preening. But it is not out of place to suggest that most of us can take some appropriate and reasonable steps to improve our appearance.

As stated above, heredity largely determines what we look like. We can, through intense exercise and extreme self-discipline, change our muscular appearance and even our posture when we are in our youth, but without consistent effort and attention these changes may not be evident as we age. Appearance *can* be changed, but it takes constant attention to proper exercise and nutrition to maintain such changes.

WEIGHT TRAINING PROGRAMS FOR FITNESS AND DEFINITION

Everytime you see or hear of a recommended exercise program, it includes a caution that you make certain you are in good health before you begin exercising. These cautions are very good advice! The older you are, the more important it is to check with your doctor before you start. (However, anyone could benefit from a *good* checkup.)

The following exercise programs are provided to help you set up an exercise routine. They are presented in a generally less-stressful to more-stressful order. The bodybuilding routines require similar energy expenditure. (All of the exercises in the following weight training routines are illustrated in Chapter Seven.)

This program requires a workout three days per week—MWF or TThS. The exercises are done in circuits, which means that the exerciser completes one set of each exercise in the circuit, then the second set of each exercise is done rather than doing two sets of one exercise in succession.

Fitness Program 1

	Exercise	Sets	Reps
	Curl	2	6-10
	Tricep press	2	6-10
Circuit these exercises	Bench press	2	6-10
	Leg extension	2	6-10
	Leg curl	2	6-10
Circuit these exercises	Pullups	2	6-10
	Lat. pulldown	2	6-10
	Situps, bent knee	2	20-30
	Jog, swim, or cycle for 15–20 minutes		

Fitness Program 2

(This program is more difficult than 1.)

Exercise	Dosage
Day 1	
Bench press	First three workouts, do 3 sets of your 10RM. Thereafter, 3 sets of your 8RM; rest 2-3 minutes between sets.
Incline dumbbell press (Superset with dumbbell flies)	Same set-rep routine as the bench press. Superset means follow immediately without resting. Do 1 set of inclines then 1 set of flies. Repeat 3 times.
Incline dumbbell curls (Superset with standing barbell curls)	Same workout as bench press.

Fitness Program 2 (continued)

Exercise	Dosage

Day 1 (continued)

| Abdominal work | Leg raises, hands under hips—2 sets of 20 |
| | Situps, bent knee—2 sets of 30 |

Jog, swim, or cycle for 20 minutes

Day 2

Squats	First three workouts, do 3 sets of your 10RM; thereafter 3 sets of your 8RM. Rest 2–4 minutes between sets.
Leg extensions	3 sets of 15 reps
Leg curls	3 sets of 15 reps
Heel raises	2 sets of 20
Lying tricep presses (Superset with tricep dips)	3 sets of 8
Abdominal work	Leg raises, hands under hips—2 sets 30 reps
	Crunch situps—2 sets 40 reps

Jog, swim, or cycle for 20-25 minutes

Day 3

Deadlift	First three workouts, do 3 sets of your 10RM; thereafter three sets of your 8RM. Rest 2–4 minutes between sets.
Pullups	3 sets of 10
Bent over rowing (Superset with lat pulldown)	3 sets of 10
Bent arm pullovers	3 sets of 10

Abdominal work:

| Leg Raises | 3 phase (1 left side, 1 center, 1 right side), 2 sets of 10 each (30 reps) |
| Crunch Situps | 2 sets of 50 |

Jog, swim, or cycle for 20–25 min.

Day 4, repeat day 1

Day 5, repeat day 2

Day 6, repeat day 3

Day 7, rest

Bodybuilders plan workouts according to body parts. The body parts normally included in the routine are shoulders, biceps, triceps, forearms, chest, back, abdominals, thighs, and calves. A workout for neck muscles is also often included.

Definition Routine

Some points to remember about a definition routine are the following:

1. You should not go on this routine until you have bulked up to a good size.
2. The best type of definition training is hard and fast, with no more than 30 seconds rest between exercises. Working in this manner requires you to reduce the weight for various exercises.
3. Pick four exercises for each body part. Do four or five sets.
4. Use this program for six to eight weeks before a contest.

The following is an example of a six-day-per-week definition routine.

Monday-Wednesday-Friday

Chest	Set	Reps
Incline press	5	10
Dips	5	15
Pulley flies	5	10
Pullovers (bent arm)	5	15
Lats	Set	Reps
Wide grip chins	5	10–12
Seated cable rowing	5	10
Lat. machine pulldowns	5	10
One-arm rowing	5	10–12
Legs	Set	Reps
Front squats	5	10–12
Hack squats	5	15
Leg extensions	5	15
Leg curls	5	15
Calf machine	6	20
Donkey calf raises	6	20

Tuesday-Thursday-Saturday

Shoulders (deltoids)	Set	Reps
Dumbbell press	5	10
Side lateral raises	5	10
Bent over lateral raises	5	12

Tuesday-Thursday-Saturday

Shoulders (deltoids)	Set	Reps
Upright rowing	4	10
Side incline raises	4	10

Biceps	Set	Reps
Incline curls	5	8-10
Bent over barbell curls	5	10
Seated dumbbell curls	5	10
Concentration curls	5	12

Triceps	Set	Reps
One-arm extensions (machine)	4	10
Lying tricep kickbacks	5	10
Tricep Pressdowns (lat. machine)	5	10
Lying dumbbell tricep press	5	10
Close grip tricep pressdown	4	20-30

REFERENCES

1. Kraemer, W., et al., 1990 Hormonal and growth-factor responses to heavy-resistance exercise protocols. *Journal of Applied Physiology* 69: 1442–1450.

2. Matveyev, L. 1981. *Fundamentals of Sport Learning* (trans. Albert P. Zdornykh). Moscow: Progress Publishers.

3. Selye, H. 1974. *Stress without Distress.* New York: Lippincott.

4. Sheldon, W. H., C. W. Dupertius, and E. McDermott. 1954. *Atlas of Men— A Guide for Somatotyping the Adult Male at All Ages.* New York: Harper.

5. Stone, M. H., H. O'Bryant, J. Garhammer, et al. 1982. A theoretical model of strength training. *National Strength and Conditioning Association Journal* 35: 36–39.

CHAPTER FIVE

High-Level Strength Training for Athletes and Competitive Lifters

You enter a high school weight room. About thirty-five young men are there and one adult, a coach. On the center lifting platform stands a person about six feet tall, 170-175 pounds preparing to do a deadlift. The bar is loaded to 470 pounds. The lifter carefully positions his feet. For a moment the murmuring in the background stops; all attention now centers on the lifter in knowledgeable anticipation of the stress he is about to endure. He positions his hands, chalked for better gripping, precisely on the bar. The silence is broken by one who intones rather gently but with compelling strength, "C'mon, Dave, let's get it." The lifter drops his rear, drives up with his legs, and pulls with his back. He strains for fully 2 seconds before the bar moves, then the weight clears the floor. Everyone in the room is shouting encouragement at this point "Pull, pull, pull that—keep it going!" "Don't let it beat you!" "Make it! Go! Go! Go!" The lifter has tried 1 rep. maximum deadlifts before, but the exact feelings of the incredible stress dim from one time to the next. Now he is staggered by the phenomenal effort required just to get the weight off the floor. He doesn't know if his back is going to break, or his eyes burst from their sockets, or what, but he keeps pulling and the bar inches up his lower legs to his knees.

Figure 5–1
High school
weight room

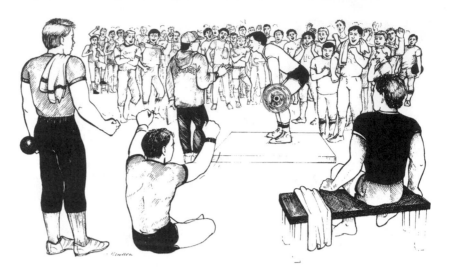

Dave's primary sticking point was getting the weight off the floor, but he does have a secondary sticking point just above his knees. Ordinarily it is no big problem, but considering how much energy and effort it took to get the bar to his knees, will he be able to go through it? Neither Dave nor anyone else in the room knows. The bar hits the stick point, Dave bends back and throws back his head, mouth open, straining with everything he has. The place is a madhouse now: "Keep pulling, now is when you find out what you are made of!" "Go, Dave!" "All the way!" "Drive your hips up and forward," shouts his coach. The bar is sliding ever so slightly up his thighs. Dave, struggling with all his might, still has his head back and knees bent. His face is red, the grimace shows his stress, ample evidence of the tremendous test he is undergoing, and there is some uncertainty there. His coach sees the uncertainty and thinks, "This is just right. The boy was supposed to try a weight that he was not certain of lifting and that is exactly what he has done." "C'mon, Dave, beat it, don't drop it!" "Let's go!" Since the bar hit the stick point it has moved about one inch up Dave's thighs. Everyone continues to cheer, but now Dave's hands start to open. "Don't drop it, Dave!" "Hang on, Man!" "Hang on and Pull!" When those in the room perceive his hands opening, the intensity of their encouragement picks up, they cheer and plead, but Dave has given his all.

His hands open, the bar drops, Dave staggers back. His coach grabs him in a semi-embrace, "Great effort, Dave!" "You'll make that lift next time." One month later, to the screaming, cheering, back-pounding glee of his teammates, Dave makes the 470 deadlift.

The scene just described could happen in any of thousands of high schools, colleges, or universities around the United States. Strength training for athletes in many sports has become almost as important as the practice of the sport itself.

Maximum lift days, when athletes lay it on the line, are competitive tests that can be intense and important sessions to both the athletes and coaches. They should not be scheduled too frequently! Once every two months for a particular lift is adequate.

The objective of the strength training discussed in Chapters Three and Four is strength fitness for toning and shaping the physique. The objective of the strength training discussed in this chapter is the development of maximum strength and human power.

WHAT DETERMINES A PERSON'S STRENGTH LEVEL?

Strength is one's ability to apply force. This force can be isometric, concentric, or eccentric. Generally, the following factors determine one's strength at any point in time:

1. The number of motor units that respond to the stimulus. The more motor units involved, the stronger the contraction. (Training can improve this.)
2. The rate of firing of motor units. Muscle tension increases as the frequency of the stimulus and the rate of firing increases. (Training can improve this.)
3. Synchronization of motor units. This simultaneous firing of many motor units produces great waves of force at very high strength stress levels. (Training *probably* can improve this.)
4. The timing of the motor unit firing and muscle contraction. Coordination of movement is essential for success in any activity. Coordinated force production produces greater force (strength) than otherwise. (Training can improve this.)
5. Inhibition, both nervous and psychological. Subconscious protective mechanisms limit maximal force output, and most human beings have some aversion to trying maximal lifts without thorough preparation. (Training can improve this.)
6. Fiber types. Fast glycolytic and fast oxidative-glycolytic muscle fibers contract faster, with greater force output, than slow twitch fibers. (There may be some potential to increase the number of fast twitch fibers.)
7. The amount of muscle mass. There is a high correlation between muscle cross sectional area and muscular force output. (Training can improve this.)
8. Anatomical attachments of tendons and the shape of the skeleton. The attachment of the tendons on the lever system (skeleton) and

the resultant angles of pull determine the ultimate potential to produce force. (Training cannot change these characteristics.)

9. A person's age. After about age thirty-five the maximal strength of most people gradually decreases. Individuals of the same chronological age may be dramatically different in terms of physical age.

Note all of the factors listed above are influenced by a person's heredity and physical condition.

HOW SHOULD ATHLETES STRENGTH TRAIN?

High-Level Strength Training

There are some exceptions for some sports, but in most cases athletes should engage in what I refer to as high-level strength training (HLST). High-level strength training is the name I give to a strength training system that has, as its *core,* some combination of the following exercises: squats, stepups, lunges (leg thrusting); bench presses, incline presses, push presses (pushes or presses); and deadlifts, cleans, high pulls, or snatches (pulls). Notice that all are free-weight, large muscle-mass, multisegment (more than one joint) exercises. When athletes perform, the entire body works in space performing any number of complex movements. Lifting free weights in space, has greater functional application to athletic movement than pushing or pulling on a resistance that is directionally controlled by a track on a machine. In most cases, effective athletic participation requires repeated explosive power output combined with careful neuromuscular control. Many of the exercises in HLST require precisely those characteristics. Plyometric exercise, another form of athletic conditioning emphasizing explosive movement, which should also be included in athletic conditioning, is discussed later in this chapter.

Basic Principles of High-Level Strength Training

1. *Total volume* means the total amount of weight lifted based on resistance level (weight), sets, repetitions, and frequency of workout in a period of time (day, week, month, year, or several years). Total volume can be approximated by counting the number of repetitions completed and multiplying by an assumed average resistance for each repetition.

2. *Frequency* refers to the number of exercise sessions participated in per day, week, or month. *Duration* can refer to the time spent in any one workout or to the length of time in a training cycle. Neither of these characteristics of an exercise routine is meaningful if the intensity (see below) of each training session is not able to be measured.

3. *Intensity,* or the rate of doing work. Intensity can be described as the number of repetitions completed at a particular weightload in a particular unit of time (the power output). The greater the power output per unit of time, the greater the intensity. Increasing one's maximum potential power output is the desired outcome of HLST. High-level strength training requires that a person do what is known as *high force exercise.* High force exercise can mean three things: (1) resistance at 80 to 100 percent of the 1RM. The speed of movement when lifting a resistance this heavy is necessarily slow or, in the case of some very powerful individuals, possibly moderate. (2) High speed exercise, characterized by relatively light weight (40 to 70 percent of the 1RM) at high movement speed, (3) A combination of the two. Fast twitch fibers are responsible for high power output (1, 2, 3, 5, 7, 8). Logically, therefore, activities that challenge or improve fast twitch fibers enhance human power. High-level strength training, properly designed, produces this effect. Intensity can be estimated by calculating the total amount of weight lifted in the time spent working out (/day, /week, /month, etc.) Intensity is normally maximized during the latter stages of a periodized workout routine.

4. The concept of *specificity* suggests that we should practice specifically that which we want to improve. In the ultimate sense a basketball player must play basketball to get better at basketball. But is that all? Are there other activities that are specific to basketball other than playing basketball? Indeed there are. Many conditioning activities are physiologically and/or biomechanically specific to various sports. For example, we need power in most sports, and we can improve our potential to produce power in a weight room or through plyometric exercise.

If a beginner plays basketball, his or her ability to produce power in the game will improve. However, if this same beginner also engages in a strength training program his or her potential for producing power in time, will normally be even greater.

SPECIFICITY OF STRENGTH TRAINING

Developing resistive exercises that *simulate particular skilled movements* (biomechanical specificity) is an area fraught with uncertainty. Successful execution of skilled movements in sport requires fine motor coordination. Increasing the resistance in such movements may indeed strengthen the muscles doing the work, but what effect will such extra resistance have on the finely controlled firing of the motor units? After many years of experience, it is my opinion that *some* resistance exercises that imitate specific sport skills *may* have limited merit, particularly in sports requiring great power; for example, doing resisted vertical jumps to enhance driving off the line in football. However, if we were to carry this concept to the extreme we might consider requiring a basketball team to use a ball weighted to be one-fourth heavier than the regular ball; a tennis or table tennis player to play with a racquet one-fourth heavier than the normal one; or a pool player to use a one-third heavier cue. The long-term effects of this method of resistance training are not known, but principles of motor learning suggest that the results would not be good. A year of training with the heavier implements would undoubtedly produce problems in coordinating movement with the lighter equipment. *Thus specificity training is useful as long as we do not disrupt fine motor coordination with inappropriate resistance training.*

I believe that strength/power should be developed in the weight room by engaging in exercises for the *physiological* characteristics that can be identified and improved, without specifically challenging the fine motor skills necessary for success in the game.

WEIGHT TRAINING AND NEUROMUSCULAR SENSITIVITY (TOUCH)

Does weight training dull the sensitivity a person must have when making highly skilled movements like shooting a basketball, hitting a tennis or golf ball, or pitching a baseball? There is no question that the *acute* effects of a weight training workout on fine motor coordination can be quite negative. Go through an intense workout of curls, tricep presses, lat. pulldowns, and bench presses, then, within 1 minute after finishing, try to shoot a basketball! A person's ability to do this immediately after intense weight training is usually quite poor. However, after a few minutes of overcoming the acute effects of weight training and loosening up, most people experience a return to normal, and some even go through a period of heightened neuromuscular control. They shoot with uncanny accuracy. The only study done on this question shows no negative effects of strength training on coordination (6).

Athletes can also lose their touch by overtraining and becoming stale. *Variety in the training program*, to include different exercises, modalities, and training load, can help athletes train without such consequences. A primary objective of periodized conditioning programs is to avoid staleness (9).

STRENGTH AND PERFORMANCE

Not all people respond in the same way to a weight training program, but all who persist get stronger. It can be stated with relative accuracy that *most* sports require a relatively high degree of strength. Once that strength level is achieved, additional strength has little effect on improving performance. A strength profile required for reasonably high level achievement in any given sport could be developed by coaches and athletes involved in the game. For example, a football lineman or shotputter must have much greater absolute strength levels than a golfer; however, a golfer must also have a relatively high strength level to be successful. *Until athletes achieve adequate strength levels for their chosen sport, they cannot be successful at the highest levels.*

The following strength profile of a world class male discus thrower is an example of strength needed for success in this particular sport. Notice that there is a range of strength in the profile. However, even the lower levels are representative of significant strength achievement.

Bench press	360–500 (lbs)
Squat (parallel)	550–700 (lbs)
Clean	360–450 (lbs)
Snatch	260–330 (lbs)
Deadlift	600–720 (lbs)

Some athletes are genetically blessed with more strength/power than others. They do not have to struggle as intensely in weight rooms to gain the strength necessary to be effective in competition. Those who don't have great genetic strength benefit more from strength training than their gifted peers. However, *there are simply too many variables in the "good-athlete" equation to suggest that if athletes gain more strength they are then going to become significantly better athletes.* Converting strength gained in the weight room to improved performance on the field is not a one-for-one proposition for most of us. It is not uncommon for the strongest person on a team not to be among the starters; however, neither is it uncommon for the strongest person to also be among the best.

STRENGTH TRAINING PROGRAMS FOR ATHLETES

Proper rest and/or recovery between sets and exercise is critical to the success of any strength training routine. In the set-rep routines of high-level strength training, after the preparation phase and exclusive of warmup sets, the recovery time between sets will be between 2 and 5 minutes. Lifters who work in groups of three will have about 3 minutes between sets. This rest is appropriate because when an athlete begins each set, he or she should feel rested, not fatigued. *Resting too short a time between sets is not conducive to maximal strength development.* Certainly a person can rest too long between sets; two to five minutes is normally adequate for most lifters.

Sets, repetitions, and weight are noted using a three number sequence, as follows: 2-4-70 percent. This sequence would mean 2 sets of 4 repetitions, with 70 percent of a person's 1 repetition maximum.

Illustrations of the following exercises can be found in Chapter Seven. The set-repetition sequences that follow can be used for bench presses, squats, incline presses, lunges, and deadlifts.

Workout Routine 1	Workout Routine 2	Workout Routine 3
1–8–40%	1–8–40%	1–8–40%
1–6–60%	1–6–60%	1–6–60%
5–5–80%	1–5–80%	3–4–80%
	1–4–90%	2–2–90%
	1–5–80%	1–6–70%

The following examples of workout routines show total poundage lifted when each repetition is counted, assuming that the 1RM for the lift is 300.

Routine (SQ-BP-DL)	Time to Complete	Total Weight Lifted (lbs)
1–8–50% (150)	26 minutes	6420
3–4–80% (240)		
2–2–90% (270)		
1–6–70% (210)		
1–6–50% (150)	23 minutes	6900
5–5–80% (240)		
1–6–60% (180)	20 minutes	6180
1–6–80% (240)		
1–2–90% (270)		
1–6–80% (240)		
1–8–70% (210)		

The clean, snatch, and high-pull workouts are characterized by fewer repetitions at what I refer to as the significant stress levels—60 percent of the 1RM and above. Some examples follow:

Routine 1	Routine 2	Routine 3
1–5–40%	1–5–40%	1–5–40%
1–3–60%	1–3–60%	1–3–60%
1–3–70%	4–3–75%	1–2–80%
1–2–80%		1–1–90%
1–5–60%		1–2–80%
1–5–60%		1–3–70%

    Following are two examples of snatch, clean, and high-pull routines with specific weight, time, and total weight lifted, assuming 1RM is 200 pounds.

Routine-(snatch, clean, hi-pull)	Time to Complete (approx.)	Total Weight Lifted (lbs.)
1–5–50% (100)	21 minutes	1880
1–3–60% (120)		
1–3–70% (140)		
1–2–80% (160)		
1–3–70% (140)		
1–3–60% (120)		
1–5–50% (100)	27 minutes	3000
1–3–60% (120)		
2–3–70% (140)		
3–3–80% (160)		
1–3 60% (120)		

    Now here is a periodized seven-week athlete workout program (core lifts only).

Monday	Wednesday	Friday
Week 1		
Bench press		
3–10–60%	3–10–70%	2–1–70%
2–10–65%		2–10–75%
Squats		
3–10–60%	3–10–75%	3–10–70%
2–10–65%		2–10–73%
Cleans		
3–6–70%	3–6–75%	2–6–65%
	2–6–65%	2–6–70%
Week 2		
Bench press		
3–10–70%	3–10–75%	2–10–70%
2–10–73%		2–10–75%
Squats		
3–10–70%	3–10–75%	2–10–73%
2–10–73%		2–10–78%
Cleans		
3–6–73%	3–6–68%	2–6–65%
	2–6–73%	2–6–73%

Monday	Wednesday	Friday
Week 3		
Bench press		
3–8–75%	3–8–80%	2–8–75%
2–8–77%		2–8–80%
Squats		
3–8–75%	3–8–80%	2–8–75%
2–8–77%		2–8–80%
Cleans		
3–4–75%	3–4–73%	2–4–73%
	2–4–75%	2–4–80%
Week 4 (Active Rest)		
Play games (1 hour):	Test 1RM	Test 1RM in
Basketball, racquetball	in Squat and Bench	Deadlift
tennis, and/or soccer	Press; play games	Play games
Week 5		
12-inch box stepups (percentages are of squat 1RM)		
2–6–50%	3–6–53%	3–6–58%
2–6–55%		
Incline press (percentages are of bench press 1RM)		
2–6–60%	3–6–65%	3–6–63%
2–6–65%		
High pulls (percentages are of clean 1RM)		
3–4–90%	2–5–80%	3–6–75%
	2–5–85%	
Week 6		
12-inch box stepups		
2–5–60%	3–5–60%	2–5–58%
2–5–63%		2–5–60%
Incline press		
2–4–67%	3–4–63%	2–4–65%
2–4–70%		2–4–67%
High pulls		
3–3–90%	3–4–80%	3–3–95%
Week 7		
Squats	High pulls	Squats
3–2–90%	3–3–90%	3–3–88%
Bench press	12-inch box stepups	Bench press
3–2–95%	2–5–65%	3–3–90%
Cleans	Incline press	Cleans
3–3–88%	2–4–67%	3–2–90%

PLYOMETRIC WORK

When we discuss speed of movement remember that we are ultimately referring to the power of the athlete. Strength training for athletes is used primarily as a means of improving physical power.

The 1980s saw the introduction and general acceptance of plyometrics. The purpose of plyometric work is essentially the same as that of strength training: to develop greater physical power (quickness). The basic physiological concept is to rapidly put the muscle under stress, stretch (shock the muscle), and then rebound with a strong concentric contraction as quickly as possible.

The legs and hips have been the major focus of plyometric exercises, with somewhat less emphasis placed on the arms and shoulders. The classic plyometric movement is to step off a height into space, arrest downward movement as quickly as possible on landing, and then explode upward with a violent concentric contraction. The initial height from which an exerciser should step out into space and allow gravity to accelerate his or her body to the landing surface should be low. The height can be moved up as a person becomes conditioned to the work. Most athletes start at a height of one foot and progressively increase, up to a maximum of about 18 to 22 inches. Of course, some athletes have gone higher, but I do not recommend that you do so. The potential for injury increases as the height increases. Coaches and athletes need to use reasonable caution when starting a plyometric program!

A common plyometric setup would include five or six sturdy wooden boxes in a properly spaced series. Athletes would be instructed to bound through the series three to six times.

Today athletes may do a number of different plyometric jumping or bounding drills as an aid in developing power. Single-leg repetitive jumps, double-leg repetitive jumps, repetitive jumps over hurdles, triple jumps, quadruple jumps, and the classic jumping from different height boxes (depth jumping).

Plyometric work for the upper limbs is not as easy to design as for the legs and hips, but there are some recommended activities. Two athletes tossing a medicine ball back and forth in a variety of ways and at varying velocities produces the shocking (catching) stretching and throwing (rebounding) effect desired. Doing pushups in a violent, drive-yourself-off-the-floor, fall back, catch, and rebound-off-the-floor movement is also plyometric in nature. Pushups or arm-bounding off walls or tables would also be plyometric work for the upper limbs. A weight training/conditioning program for athletes without plyometric exercise would be missing an important ingredient.

COMPETITIVE LIFTING

The discussions in previous sections have presented strength training as a means to an end (body shaping, speed, quickness, power) but not as an objective in and of itself. In this section, we consider those whose objective is to lift weights: competitive weightlifters and powerlifters.

All who strive mightily, in whatever field, are characterized by certain similarities. Most willingly and joyfully devote a large amount of time to their activity, time passed in doing that which expresses their personhood more completely and uniquely than perhaps any other activity. Such individuals are at least somewhat obsessed with their chosen pursuit. Time spent pursuing their goals is not thought of as a sacrifice by these athletes, even though when awards are won and speeches are given there is the inevitable reference to the great sacrifice required to get to a certain level of athletic achievement. Let the speechmakers pontificate. Athletes know that the real sacrifice in their lives is giving up training and competing to do something else life requires of them. For most who are engaged in competitive lifting, there is an attraction to what they do that is quite beyond explanation. The activity is so much a part of their being that statements such as "I enjoy that," or "I am intrigued by that," or "I love that," are quite inadequate.

These people passionately chase something that may bring them glory, fame, money, and self-satisfaction. It may also bring them disappointment, defeat, social dereliction, and/or poverty. Of no one is this narrative more descriptive than the world class athlete. Enraptured devotion does not describe all Olympic lifters and powerlifters but it does describe the very best.

Olympic Weightlifting

There are two forms of competitive lifting. The older is known as Olympic lifting, and the more recent is powerlifting. Some form of weightlifting has been contested in the Olympic Games since their modern rebirth in 1896. The Olympic lifts contested today, the *two-hands snatch* and the *two-hands clean and jerk,* were initiated in the 1932 Olympic Games. The two-hands clean and overhead press was an Olympic lift from 1932 until 1972. In 1972 the press was eliminated because it had basically evolved into another overhead jerk.

The two Olympic lifts are often referred to as the *quick lifts* because their successful execution requires that the lifter move very quickly during certain phases of the lifts. Successful Olympic lifters are among the most powerful of athletes (4). Their task in both lifts is to move hundreds of pounds from the floor to arm's length overhead. To accomplish the two lifts, these athletes must be very flexible and quickly apply great power with precise timing and balance. It has always struck me that there is no more demanding activity in all of sport than Olympic lifting. When competing, the task of Olympic lifters is to lift as much as possible, not 85 or 95 percent but the absolute maximum, with the greatest possible speed and precise balance. Massive weight, great speed (violent motion), and the requirement for precise balance—nothing can be more complex.

Techniques of Olympic Weightlifting
The Two-Hands Snatch (Squat Style) (See Figure 5–2.)

For this lift the hook grip is used. In the hook grip, the first and second fingers are wrapped *over* the thumb. This grip enables a lifter to hold more weight than is otherwise possible. A good way to determine initial grip width on the bar for a snatch lift is to extend the arms laterally from the shoulders, then bring the forearms to a vertical position, elbows forming a right angle. Measure the distance between the forefingers, and use this measurement for initial grip width. Experiment with wider and narrower grips to determine which feels best.

The starting position. (See A.) Feet 6 to 12 inches apart (usually not more than 10 in.), toes turned slightly out, the bar directly over the joint where the big toe joins the foot (metatarsal-phalangeal joint). The lifter assumes a squat position over the bar, back flat, shins very near the bar, the hips quite low. The hips may be at the same elevation as the knees or slightly higher. Experimentation determines the best position for each individual.

The pull. The pull can be initiated from a stationary position or with a bobbing up and down of the hips. The *first phase* of the pull (See B.) is initiated by the strong muscles of the legs and hips contracting to drive the hips upward. When the bar reaches knee height the angle between the

Figure 5-2
Two-hands snatch

A. Starting position

B. End of first phase, beginning of second phase of pull

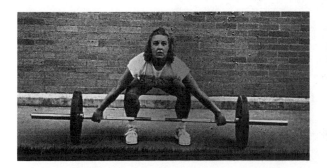
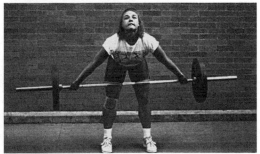

C. End of second phase of pull

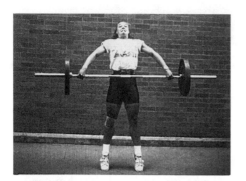

D. Squat position

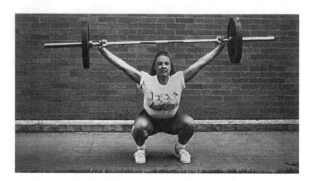

back and the lifting platform should be essentially the same as it was when the pull began. The arms remain straight, the shoulders forward, and the shins vertical. The *second phase* of the pull (See C.) begins as the bar passes the knees. The hips are driven forward and upward, and the shoulders are pulled up and slightly back as the erector muscles of the back contract forcefully. The chest and head are also lifted, to assist in imparting speed and height to the bar. The lifter should rise on the balls of his or her feet at this time. Arms are still straight. The *third phase* of the pull begins as the body is fully extended. This phase includes only a shoulder shrug and a bending of the elbows as the bar is raised to chest level. At this point the lifter very quickly drops into a low squat position (See D.) twisting the wrists under the bar and locking the elbows. After gaining balance in the squat position, the lifter must come to an erect standing position with the bar overhead and hold that position for a moment (See E). Precise timing and balance, combined with very good flexibility, are required for the successful execution of this lift.

E. Finishing position

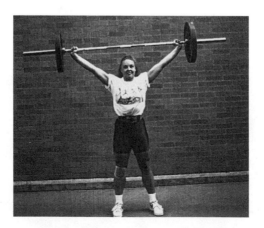

Figure 5–3
Two-hands clean

A. Starting position

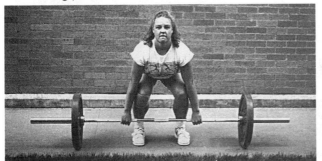

B. Finish of the pull phase

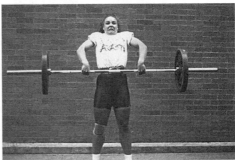

The Two-Hands Clean and Jerk
Clean Phase (See Figure 5–3.)

    The starting position. (See A.) The hands are placed on the bar a little wider than shoulder width using the hook grip described for the snatch. The feet are spaced hip-width apart (the outside edge of the heels perpendicular to the outside edge of the hips) or a little less. The bar should be directly over the metatarsal joint of the great toes. The feet may be turned out slightly. The lifter assumes a squat position, the back should be flat, and the hips at knee height or lower. The trunk is relatively upright and the arms straight.

    The pull. (See B.) The pull is initiated by a powerful upward drive of the hips and legs. The back should maintain very close to the same angle as in the start position until the bar passes the knees. Shoulders remain over the bar. When the bar is at knee height, the shins are vertical, arms straight. The second phase of the pull begins as the bar passes the knees. The hips are thrust forward and upward as the back violently extends. The bar brushes the thighs, moves slightly forward, and passes the hips as

C. Catch or racked position

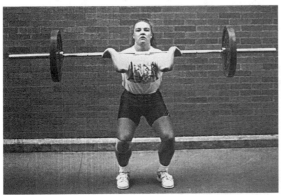

D. Clean position; beginning of the jerk

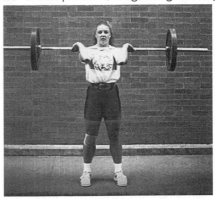

Figure 5–3 Two-Hands Clean *(continued)*

E. Split jerk

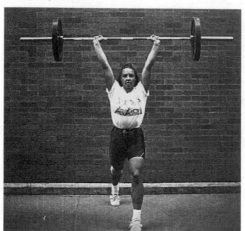

F. Finishing position

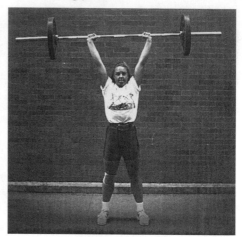

the lifter rises on the balls of the feet. The body fully extends, the shoulders shrug, and the elbows bend upward. From this fully extended position, with the bar at waist height or slightly above, the lifter drops very quickly to a deep front squat position. As the elbows are rotated from above the bar to a position in front of and below the bar, the wrists rotate the bar on its axis to facilitate this action. The bar is "racked" on the hands, deltoids, and clavicles (See C). The lifter then rises to an upright position. This action is best accomplished by not stopping at all in the low squat position.

The Jerk phase. (See D.) Once the lifter is in the upright position with the bar racked on the shoulders, he or she unhooks the thumbs and grips the bar in a normal pronated grip. The lifter then drops into a very shallow squat, rebounds vigorously from this position, and drives the bar violently upward off the shoulders and chest. At about the time the bar is passing the chin or lips, the lifter "splits" his legs front and back (not side to side) and drops quickly under the bar (See E). Which leg goes forward and which goes back is a matter of personal preference. The weight is taken on the flat front foot and the ball of the rear foot The feet should be pointing straight forward or turned slightly outward. The combined overhead thrust and drop into the split position help the lifter fully extend the arms and lock the elbows. The lifter recovers to an upright position by bringing the front foot back under the hips and then bringing the rear foot forward. When both the body and bar are immobile, the lift has been successfully completed (See F).

Powerlifting

Techniques of Powerlifting

The lifts in competitive powerlifting are the parallel squat, the bench press, and the deadlift. The technique descriptions that follow are purposely relatively brief. Their purpose is merely to introduce you to powerlifting.

The Parallel Squat. (See Figure 5–4.) While the bar is still in the squat rack, it is precisely balanced on the lifter's back, not more than one inch below the top of the deltoid muscles (See A). The lowest possible position of the bar on the back is a mechanical advantage. Lifting rules allow only one inch below the top of the deltoid muscles. Once the lifter has taken the weight off the rack he or she steps backward away from the rack. The lifter can position the feet at any width of stance that feels the strongest. Most lifters use a stance shoulder-width apart or slightly more, with the feet slightly turned out (5–10°). Once the lifter has taken a stance he or she waits for the referee's signal. When the referee signals by saying "Squat," the lifter squats down, keeping the knees over the toes, to a depth deep enough that a line drawn from the top of the knee to the crease in the hip would break parallel with the floor (See B). The lifter then returns to the upright or erect position, at which time the lift is complete. (Reracking the bar is not part of the lift.)

The Bench press. (See Figure 5–5.) The lifter assumes a supine position on the bench. The feet must remain flat on the floor and the buttocks and shoulders must be in contact with the bench throughout the lift. The

Figure 5–4 Parallel Squat

A. Starting and finishing position

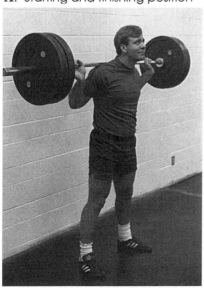

B. Squat position

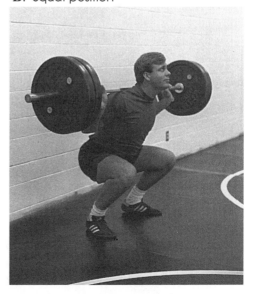

Figure 5–5
Bench Press

A. Starting and finishing position

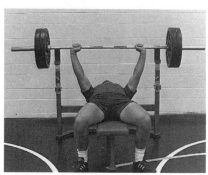

B. Pause position

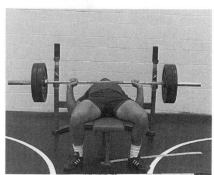

lifter takes a pronated grip on the bar with a maximum width between the forefingers of 81 centimeters, or 31 7/8 inches. A spotter usually helps the lifter get the bar to arms' length above his or her chest. When the spotter takes his hand off the bar, the lifter lowers the bar to the chest, where it *must momentarily pause* before being pressed back up to the starting position with arms extended. The path travelled upward is normally obliquely up and back, not straight up off the chest. The oblique path is slightly easier than straight up.

The Deadlift. (See Figure 5–6.) There are two basic styles of deadlifting: one with a narrow, orthodox stance, with the arms outside the legs, and the other with a wide stance, arms inside the legs (sumo style). Deadlifters generally use an alternating grip (one hand supinated, the other pronated) to prevent the bar from spinning out of the hands. Using the *narrow stance,* the lifter stands in front of the bar with heels not more than ten inches apart toes turned out slightly, squats down, and takes a good grip (See A). The lifter then lowers the buttocks until his or her back is flat. (This position is the same as the beginning position of the clean and jerk except that the grip is alternating.) The initial pull is with the hips and legs (See B). It

Figure 5–6
Deadlift
(Orthodox
Technique)

A.
Starting Position

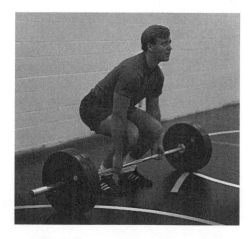

B. The midpoint, a common sticking point

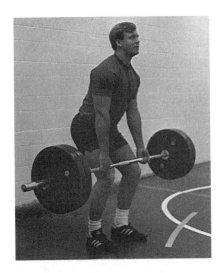

C. Finishing position

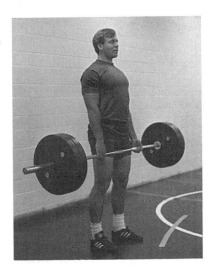

is critical that lifters lift the shoulders at the same rate as the hips. When the lifter has pulled the bar up until his or her body is erect and shoulders are back, the lift is essentially complete (See C). The rules do state, however, that the lifter must hold on to the bar as it is lowered back onto the platform. In *sumo style*, the lifter takes a wide stance in front of the bar, toes turned out at an angle of up to 45 degrees. The lifter then squats down and grips the bar. The best positioning of the hands on the bar is directly below the shoulders. Once the grip is taken, the lifter flattens the back, squats low with the legs, putting the back in a nearly vertical position. The lifter then lifts the bar until achieving an upright or erect position with the bar hanging at arm's length in front of the body.

Training Principles for Competitive Lifting

The following training concepts are very important. Use of these concepts when designing a program will result in a reasonably sound routine.

1. Consistency in training is critically important. You must be consistent or progress will be very slow or nonexistent.
2. Training loads anywhere from 50 to 100 percent of the 1RM are effective in training for Olympic lifting. Training loads for powerlifting are usually above 75 percent of the 1RM. The difficulty of a workout is determined more by the number of sets and repetitions than by how much is lifted in a given set. For example, five sets of 5 at 80 percent of the 1RM is a heavy workout. Two sets of 5 at 80 percent is a light to moderate workout.
3. Over a training cycle the workout usually varies from a lighter weight with more repetitions to a heavier weight and fewer repetitions.

4. There is no best training load for everyone. Some people obtain the best results using 75 to 80 percent of maximum others using 90 to 100 percent.

5. Some people have greater muscular endurance than others. One person may be able to do 3 repetitions at 95 percent of the 1RM, while another may only do one even if they have similar maximum lifts.

6. There is no universal, ideal workout frequency when training for the Olympic or powerlifts. A person will need to experiment with different systems to find out what is best for him.

7. Beginners can find positive results using almost any program. But the more capable a person becomes, the more carefully his or her training program(s) must be designed.

The training programs that follow are examples of routines Olympic and powerlifters might use in preparing for a competition.

Powerlifting Training Programs

Program 1: Eight-Week Cycle, 3 Days per Week

Objectives are to add five pounds per week to the bench press reps and ten pounds per week for the squat and deadlift. At midcycle, back off to one half the gains and start again.

The following program is based on a beginning strength levels of 353 pounds for the bench press, 470 pound deadlift, and a 468 pound squat.

Monday	Wednesday	Friday
Week 1		
Heavy Bp 5x5 start at 80%-85% of max (300 lb)	Heavy DL 3x5-85% max (400 lb) 2x2-95% max (450)	Moderate Squat 3x4-85% (400 lb) 1x3-95% (445)
Heavy SQ 5x5 start at 85% of max (400)	BP Moderate 2x4-80% (280) 2x2-90% (320)	BP Light 3x3-90% (320) DL Light 3x4-85% (400)
Week 2		
BP 5x5-305 SQ 5x5-410	DL 3x5-410 2x2-460 BP 2x4-28 2x2x-33	SQ 3x4-410 1x3-455 BP 3x3-325 DL 3x4-410
Week 3		
BP 5x5-310 SQ 5x5-420	DL 3x5-420 2x2-460	SQ 3x4-420 1x3-465

3021900007 2660

Monday	Wednesday	Friday
	BP 2x4-290	BP 3x3-330
	2x2x-33	DL 3x4-420

Week 4

BP 5x5-315	DL 3x5-430	SQ 3x4-430
SQ 5x5-430	2x2-480	1x3-475
	BP 2x4-295	BP 3x3-335
	2x2 -335	DL 3x4-430

Week 5

BP 5x5-305 or 310	DL 3x5-420	SQ 3x4-420
(Depends	2x2-470	1x3-465
on specifically	BP 2x4-285	BP 3x3-330
how the lifter feels)		
SQ 5x5-420	2x2-325	DL 3x4-420

Week 6

BP 5x4-320	DL 3x4-450	SQ 3x3-430
SQ 5x4-440	2x2-480	1x3-475
	BP 2x3-290	BP 3x3-330
	2x2-335	DL 3x4-430

Week 7

BP 5x3-340	DL 3x3-480	SQ 3x3-450
SQ 5x3-470	2x2-500	1x3-485
	BP 2x3-300	BP 3x3-335
	2x2-340	DL 3x4-440

Week 8

BP determine 1RM	DL determine 1RM	SQ 3x2-90%
SQ determine 1RM	BP 3x2-85%	BP 3-3-80%
		DL 3x4-85%

Program 2: Ten-Week Cycle, 4 Days per Week

Coding various set, repetition, and resistance levels helps in putting a large amount of information in a relatively small space. Below is an example of a coding system. Workouts are written by set, repetition, and percentage of 1RM. For example, 1x 8-80% would mean 1 set of 8 repetitions at 80 percent of the 1 repetition maximum.

Key to letters below:

A.	1x8-60%,	1x8-70%,	4x8-80%	
B.	1x8-60%,	1x8-70%,	2x3-80%,	2x2-90%
C.	1x8-60%,	1x6-70%,	3x5,7-80%	
D.	1x8-60%,	1x6-75%,	4x5-85%	

E. 1x8-60%, 1x6-75%,   3x5,6-85%
F. 1x8-60%, 1x5-75%,   1x5-85%,   1x3,4-90%,   2x2-90%
G. 1x8-60%, 1x4-75%,   1x4-85%,   3x3-90%
H. 1x8-60%, 1x5-75%,   1x4-85%,   1x3-90%,   2x2-95%
I. 1x8-60%, 1x5-75%,   1x3-85%,   2x2-95%
J. 1x8-60%, 1x3-75%,   1x2-85%,   1x1 new maximum

The following four-day workout includes assistance exercises for the bench press, squat, and deadlift. There are various possibilities, but I recommend the following lifts: squat assistance—heavy partial squats, or box squats, bench press assistance—weighted dips, and deadlift assistance—partial deadlifts in a rack, stiff-legged deadlifts, or deadlifts off blocks.

Monday	Wednesday	Thursday	Friday
Heavy bench	Heavy deadlift	Light bench	Light squat
Heavy squat	Deadlift assistance	Bench assistance	Squat assistance
			Light deadlift

A ten-week cycle with two competitions scheduled a month apart might look like the following:

Week	1	2	3	4	5 (Competition on Saturday)	6	7	8	9	10 (Competition on Saturday)
Monday										
BP	A	A	F	H	I	J	A	F	I	J
SQ	D	D	G	G	J	I	A	H	G	I
Wednesday										
DL	C	D	G	F	J	H	D	H	I	C
DL assistance					0					0
Thursday										
BP	C	C	B	B	C	0	B	I	B	0
BP assistance										
Friday										
SQ	E	C	C	B	C	0	C	I	B	0
SQ assistance										
DL	C	E	B	C	B	0	C	E	B	0

Note: 0 = Do not work out on that lift that day.

A Five-Week Training Program for Olympic Weightlifting

Many assistance exercises are used in this four-days-per-week program taking five weeks to complete. (Workout denotation = set, rep, percent of max. weight)

Monday	Tuesday	Thursday	Saturday
Week 1			
Power snatch	*Front squat*	*Push jerk & jerk*	*Snatch*
2x4-40%	1x5-50%	1x4-50%	1x5-50%
2x3-60%	2x5-60%	2x3-60%	1x3-70%
2x3-70%	2x5-70%	1x3-70%	5x1-82.5%
2x2-75%	3x5-80%	2x3-75%	
Push jerk & jerk			
(2 pushjerks & 1			
jerk in ea. set)	*Squat cleans*	*Jerk pressout*	*Power clean*
1x5-50%	1x4-50%	1x5-50%	1x5-50%
2x3-60%	1x3-60%	2x5-65%	2x5-60%
2x3-70%	1x3-70%	3x5-80%	2x5-65%
2x3-80%	2x2-75%		
Snatch grip	*Clean grip*		
Pressout	*deadlift*	*Snatch-high pulls*	*Back squats*
1x5-50%	1x5-60	1x5-50%	1x8-50%
2x5-60%	2x5-70%	1x4-60%	1x6-60%
2x5-70%	2x3-80%	1x3-75%	2x5-70%
3x5-75%		2x3-90%	1x5-80%
Week 2			
Push jerk & jerk	*Front squats*	*Push jerk & jerk*	*Snatch*
1x3-60%	2x5-50%	1x3-50%	1x3-50%
1x3-70%	1x5-60%	2x3-60%	2x3-60%
1x3-80%	1x5-70%	1x3-65%	1x3-70%
1x3-88%	1x5-75%	3x3-75%	2x1-80%
	3x5-85%		2x1-85%
			1x1-90%
Jerk pressouts	*Power snatch*	*Snatch grip*	*Clean and*
		pressout	*jerk*
2x5-50%	1x3-50%	1x5-50%	1x5-50%
2x5-70%	2x3-60%	2x5-60%	2x3-60%
1x5-80%	2x3-70%	3x5-70%	1x3-75%
3x5-85%			2x1-85%
			2x1-90%

Monday	Tuesday	Thursday	Saturday
Back hyper	*Snatch*		
extensions	*high pulls*		*Back Squat*
3x8 moderate	1x3-20%		1x8-60%
weight	2x3-80%		1x5-75%
	2x3-100%		2x5-80%

Week 3

Power snatch	*Front squat*	*Push jerk & jerk*	*Snatch*
1x3-50%	1x5-60%	1x3-50%	1x5-50%
1x3-55%	1x5-70%	1x3-60%	2x3-60%
1x3-60%	3x5-80%	1x3-70%	2x3-70%
1x3-65%		2x3-80%	
2x3-70%			

Push jerk & jerk	*Squat cleans*	*Clean grip pressouts*	*Clean & jerk*
1x3-50%	1x3-50%	1x5-50%	1x3-50%
1x3-55%	1x3-60%	1x5-50%	1x3-50%
1x3-60%	1x3-70%	1x5-70%	2x3-65%
1x3-65%	2x2-80%	2x5-75%	
2x3-75%			

Snatch grip pressouts	*Snatch high pulls*		*Snatch high pulls*
1x5-50%	1x3-50%		1x3-50%
1x5-60%	1x3-80%		1x3-60%
2x5-80%	2x3-90%		2x3-70%
1x5-85%			

Hyperextensions
3x8 moderate weight

Week 4

Monday	Wednesday		Saturday
Snatch	*Front squat*		*Snatch*
2x3-60%	2x5-40%		1x3-40%
2x3-70%	2x5-60%		1x3-50%
1x2-75%	1x5-70%		2x3-60%
2x1-85%	1x5-80%		2x2-70%
2x1-90%	3x5-85%		2x2-70%
1x1-95%			

Monday	Wednesday	Saturday
Clean & jerk	*Snatch High pulls*	*Clean & jerk*
1x2-75%	1x3-50%	1x3-40%
1x2-85%	1x3-60%	1x3-50%
1x1-85%	2x3-70%	1x3-60%
1x1-90%		1x3-70%
1x1-95%		2x2-75%
Clean grip	*Snatch*	*Front*
deadlift	*lockouts*	*squat*
1x5-60%	1x3-50%	1x5-40%
1x5-70%	1x3-60%	1x5-50%
2x5-80%	1x3-70%	2x3-65%
2x3-90%	1x3-80%	
	1x2-85%	
	2x2-95%	

Week 5- Contest Week

Monday	Wednesday	Saturday
1x3-40%	1x3-40%	CONTEST
1x3-50%	1x3-50%	
1x3-55%	1x3-60%	
1x3-60%	1x3-70%	
2x3-65%		
Power clean	*Power clean*	
	& jerk	
1x3-40%	1x3-40%	
1x3-50%	1x2-50%	
1x3-60%	1x2-60%	
3x2-70%	3x1-65%	
Clean grip		
pressout	*Back squat*	
1x3-50%	1x5-50%	
2x3-60%	1x5-60%	
2x3-70%	1x3-70%	
1x3-75%		

All human beings should, at some time in some activity, have the experience of giving all they have to try to become the very best they can be. Olympic and powerlifting offer that opportunity to any who may be so inclined.

REFERENCES

1. Burke, R. E., and V. R. Edgerton. 1975. Motor unit properties and selective involvement in movement. In *Exercise and Sport Sciences Reviews* (J. Wilmore and J. Keough, Eds.). New York: Academic Press.

2. Edgerton, V. R. 1976. Neuromuscular adaptation to power and endurance work. *Canadian Journal of Applied Sport Sciences* 1: 49-58.

3. Edgerton, V. R. 1978. Mammalian muscle fiber types and their adaptability. *American Zoology* 18: 113–125.

4. Garhammer, J. 1980. Power production by Olympic weightlifters. *Medicine and Science in Sport and Exercise* 12: 54–60.

5. Komi, P. V. 1979. Neuromuscular performance: Factors influencing force and speed production. *Scandinavian Journal of Sport Sciences* 1: 2—15.

6. Masley, J. W., A. Harabedian, and D. N. Donaldson. 1953. Weight training in relation to strength, speed, and coordination. *Research Quarterly* 24 (3): 308–315.

7. Maton, B. 1976. Motor unit differentiation and integrated surface EMG in voluntary isometric contraction. *European Journal of Applied Physiology* 35: 149–157.

8. Spectar, S. A., P. F. Gardiner, R. F. Zernicke, et al. 1980. Muscle architecture and force velocity characteristics of cat soleus and medial gastrocnemius: Implications for motor control. *Journal of Neurophysiology* 44: 951–960.

9. Stone, M. H., H. S. O'Bryant. 1987. *Weight Training: A Scientific Approach*. Minneapolis: Burgess.

CHAPTER SIX

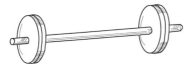

Weight Training Programs

BEGINNING A WEIGHT TRAINING PROGRAM

As you begin a weight training program you should feel pleased that you have taken a step toward improved fitness and appearance. Most of us look forward to bodily changes that make us feel and look better. We often have little appreciation of the time and effort that such changes require, but we are willing to give it a go. Improvement in physical appearance and fitness exact their toll in time and consistent effort.

A true beginner, someone who has not lifted weights before, could start lifting using almost any system and make significant strength and muscular fitness progress in a reasonably short period of time (4 to 6 weeks). There would be some soreness, and lifting very heavy weights could cause injury, but *most of us* are cautious when trying new experiences, so we tend not to overdo it. There are exceptions, however; some people injure themselves by lifting too much weight, or they become extremely sore by going through a very vigorous workout the first time they weight-train. Our bodies are really quite marvelous at adapting to new stressors, but there are limits that should not be exceeded. We should all begin weight training with a degree of restraint. It certainly is best when starting a weight training program that we seek assistance from people who know how to help us. Knowledgeable people can assist us through the awkward, potentially injurious, beginning stages of learning.

The following principles are important when beginning a program of weight training:

1. The resistance for the first two sessions should be quite light.
2. All of the major muscle groups of the body need to be exercised.
3. Rest between sets should be only long enough to recover physical working capacity—1 to 3 minutes.
4. Move the resistance (weight) through the complete range of motion—complete extension of the major movers, followed by complete flexion. Do not give in to the temptation to cut the extension phase (muscle-lengthening phase) short so that your muscles are in a stronger position to do another repetition.
5. Do not move purposely slowly nor try to move the resistance at high velocities. Move the resistance at a comfortable, "normal" cadence.
6. I recommend that you work out three times per week as a beginner in weight training. Three workouts per week have been found to be very effective for anyone interested in strength fitness. There is adequate recovery time after each workout, and the results are excellent. As you become more experienced you may choose to exercise more frequently or even less frequently. Time and motivation are primary determinants of workout frequency and length. Remember, the body is incredible at adapting to different stresses. Bodybuilders and those who compete in weightlifting may work out six to fourteen times per week Powerlifters may only lift weights twice per week during certain phases of their training cycle. Workout time and frequency is dependent on the objective(s) of the period in the training cycle.

The exercises that you as a beginner will use are no different than the exercises the more advanced lifter would use. The major differences are in the amount of weight lifted, the number of sets for each exercise, and the frequency of workout. As mentioned above, the human body adapts to any reasonable stressor if given adequate time. As you begin this program, give yourself adequate time to adjust to this new activity in your life.

It is worthwhile to make a record of your feelings as you begin this weight training program. You can easily make a few notes in your training diary. Doing so heightens your awareness of your reaction to exercise. Notice the mild soreness of the muscles. How long does it take for the soreness to go away? Are you more or less tired after a workout day? Do you sleep better when you exercise? Most people feel better about themselves when they start an exercise program; is that true for you?

The possibilities are practically limitless when it comes to writing weight training programs. Literally thousands of weight training programs could be devised by manipulating exercises, sets, repetitions, resistance levels, and workout frequencies. I have carefully selected the following weight training routines for your reference and/or use.

The beginning programs that follow are offered as very effective ways of starting on the road to strength fitness and a somewhat improved appearance. These routines are based on the assumption that the weight training facilities available are reasonably well equipped. The exercises are described in detail in Chapter Seven.

A STRENGTH FITNESS PROGRAM FOR BEGINNERS

Exercise	Muscle Group	Resistance level*	Sets/ Reps	Rest per set (minutes)
Leg Extensions	Quadriceps	10RM	3/10 RM	2–4
Leg Curls	Hamstrings	10RM	3/10 RM	2–4
Toe Presses	Calves	20RM	3/20RM	2–4
Bench Presses	Chest	10RM	3/10RM	2–4
Lat Pulldowns	Upper back	10RM	3/10RM	2–4
Upright Rowing	Shoulder	10RM	3/10RM	2–4
Triceps Pressdowns	Triceps	10RM	3/10RM	2–4
Biceps Curl	Biceps	10RM	3/10RM	2–4
Bent leg Situp	Abdominals	Bodywt.	3/30	2–4
Back hyperextensions	Lower back	Bodywt.	3/30	2–4

*The first set of each exercise should be only 70% of the 10RM weight (the weight that can be lifted just 10 times after which muscular failure occurs).

Periodized or cycled programs have gained a great deal of popularity in the past few years. Such programs produce excellent results and offer invigorating variety. The resistance levels in the different phases of the following programs are presented as a *percentage of a 1RM*. I recognize that it is difficult to determine 1RMs in all the exercises listed, and I also recognize that strength levels will change during the training cycle. However, this system of determining resistance levels is considered the most effective: therefore, the following workout routines are based on doing repetitions (sets) using percentages of the 1RM for each exercise. (The table in Chapter Two that predicts 1RM based on a set-to-failure can be used to estimate your 1RM.)

What follows is a three phase, periodized, weight training program for individuals seeking strength fitness. Each phase should include three workouts per week for a minimum of four weeks.

A THREE-PHASE, PERIODIZED, STRENGTH FITNESS PROGRAM

Phase I

The resistance levels in this *beginning* program are purposely light. A beginning lifter should start light until he or she learns the movement and becomes somewhat accustomed to the exercises. Six exercise periods (2 weeks) at the resistance levels should be adequate. After that, resistance levels should be carefully increased until at the end of 4-week cycle the exerciser should be using 10 to 15 percent more of the 1RM for each exercise.

Exercise	Muscle Group	Repetitions & Resistance level Set 1	Set 2	Set 3	Rest between Sets (minutes)
Leg extensions	Quadriceps	15/40	15/45	15/45	2–3
Leg curls	Hamstrings	15/40	15/45	15/45	2–3
Toe presses	Calves	20/50	20/55	20/55	2–3
Bench presses	Chest	12/45	12/55	12/55	2–3
Lat pulldowns	Back	12/45	12/55	12/55	2–3
Bent arm pullovers	Back	12/45	12/50	12/55	2–3
DB[1] Shrugs	Shoulders	12/45	12/55	12/55	2–3
'Seated barbell presses	Shoulders	12/45	12/50	12/50	2–3
Barbell curls	Biceps	12/45	12/50	12/55	2–3
Seated overhead triceps presses	Triceps	12/40	12/50	12/55	2–3
Bent knee situps	Abdominals	30	30	30	2
Back hyperextensions	Lower back	30	30	30	2

[1]DB=Dumbbell

Phase II

This phase is to last approximately 4 weeks. It is expected that a diligent weight trainer should be able to complete this workout, at the resistance levels listed, by the second to third week of this period. By the end of the 4 weeks the weight trainer should be able to work rapidly through the exercise routine with minimal rest between sets and exercises. This is the objective, not further increases in weight. Weight should be increased only when rest time between sets and exercises is cut to 30 seconds, and the exerciser still feels underworked!

Exercise	Muscle Group	Repetitions & Resistance level			Rest between Sets (minutes)
		Set 1	Set 2	Set 3	
Leg Presses	Quadriceps, Gluteus	10/80	10/85	10/85	3–4
Lunges	Quadriceps, Gluteus	10/60	10/70	10/75	3–4
DB[1] calf raises	Calves	25/40	25/50	25/50	3
Flat back flies	Chest	08/60	08/70	08/75	2–3
Bench presses	Chest	08/65	08/70	08/75	2–3
Good morning exercise	lower back, hamstrings	08/50	08/55	08/60	3
Seated cable row	Back	08/75	08/80	08/85	2–3
DB standing lateral raise	Shoulders	08/65	08/70	08/70	2–3
Seated DB incline curls	Biceps	08/70	08/75	08/80	2–3
Tricep pressdowns	Triceps	08/70	08/75	08/80	2–3
Crunch situps	Abdominals	20/10#	20/10#	20/10#	2–3

[1]DB=Dumbbell

Phase III

This phase is to last approximately 4 weeks. It is expected that a diligent weight trainer should be able to complete this workout, at the resistance levels listed, by the second to third week of this period. By the end of the 4 weeks the weight trainer should be able to work rapidly through the exercise routine with minimal rest between sets and exercises. That is the objective, not further increases in weight. Weight should be increased only when rest time between sets and exercises is cut to 30 seconds, and the exerciser still feels underworked!

Exercise	Muscle Group	Repetitions & Resistance Level			Rest between Sets (minutes)
		Set 1	Set 2	Set 3	
Leg presses	Quadriceps, Gluteus	08/80	08/85	06/90	3
Leg curls	Hamstrings	08/80	08/85	08/85	3
Seated calf raise	Calves	20/60	20/65	20/70	3
BB incline presses	Chest	08/80	08/80	06/85	2–3
BB narrow grip bench presses	Chest	08/70	08/75	06/80	2–3
Straight leg deadlift	Lower back, hips	08/60	08/70	06/75	3
Bent over row	Upper back	08/80	08/80	06/85	2–3
BB[1] shrugs	Trapezius	10/80	10/80	10/80	2–3
Press behind the neck, seated	Shoulders	08/70	08/75	08/80	2–3
Preacher bench curls	Biceps	08/70	08/75	06/85	2–3
Tricep pressdown	Triceps	08/80	08/85	06/90	2–3
Twisting incline situps	Abdominals	30	30	30	2
Vertical hang kneeups	Abdominals	20	25	30	2–3

BB = Barbell

A MODERATELY DEMANDING BODYBUILDING PROGRAM

A lifter who has never experienced weight training at the intensity level suggested for this workout will probably not be able to follow the time schedule recommended. However, after about 3 weeks of work (9 workouts) the pace should be able to be maintained.

Exercise	Muscle Group	Resistance Level	Sets/ Reps	Rest per Set (minutes)
Hip sleds	Quadriceps, Hamstrings	10 RM	4/10	1–2
Leg extensions	Quadriceps	10 RM	4/10	1–2
Leg curls	Hamstrings	10 RM	4/10	1–2
Bench presses	Chest	10 RM	4/10	1–2
Supine lat. raises	Chest	10 RM	4/10	1–2
Lat. pulldowns	Back	10 RM	4/10	1–2

Exercise	Muscle Group	Resistance Level	Sets/ Reps	Rest per Set (minutes)
DB bent rowing	Back	10RM	4/10	1–2
Standing DB lat raises	Shoulders	10 RM	4/10	1–2
DB overhead presses	Shoulders	10RM	4/10	1–2
Triceps pressdowns	Triceps	10RM	4/10	1–2
Seated overhead triceps presses	Triceps	10RM	4/10	1–2
DB curls	Biceps	10RM	4/10	1–2
Preacher bench curls	Biceps	10 RM	4/10	1–2
Curl-ups	Abdominals	5-15 lb.	4/20–40	1–2
Incline knee-ups	Abdominals	Bodywt.	2/50	1–2

DB=Dumbbell

A sample *periodized, three-phase weight training program for those* wanting a good combination of strength and hypertrophy follows. (Resistance levels are listed as a percentage of the 1RM for each exercise.)

A THREE-PHASE, PERIODIZED, STRENGTH-HYPERTROPHY PROGRAM

Phase I

Exercise	Muscle Group	Repetitions & Resistance Level*			Rest between Sets (minutes)
		Set 1	Set 2	Set 3	
Leg presses	Quadriceps, Hamstrings	12/60	12/70	12/75	1–2
Leg extensions	Quadriceps	12/60	12/70	12/75	1–2
Leg curls	Hamstrings	12/60	12/70	12/75	1–2
Bench presses	Chest	10/65	10/75	10/80	1–2
DB incline presses	Chest	10/65	10/75	10/80	1–2
Wide grip pullups	Back	10	12	14	1–2
Reverse grip Lat Pull	Back	10/70	10/75	10/80	1–2
Barbell Shrugs	Trapezius	10/70	10/75	10/80	1–2
BB press behind neck	Shoulders	10/65	10/70	10/75	1–2
Preacher curls	Biceps	10/65	10/70	10/75	1–2
Tricep pressdowns	Triceps	10/65	10/70	10/75	1–2
Crunch situps	Abdominals	30	40	50	1–2

Phase II

Exercise	Muscle Group	Repetitions & Resistance Level*			Rest between Sets (minutes)
		Set 1	Set 2	Set 3	
Lunges	Hip, thigh	8/70	8/75	8/80	2–3
Leg extensions	Quadriceps	8/80	8/80	8/85	1–2
Toe presses	Calves	20 RM	20 RM	20RM	1–2
Bench presses	Chest	8/75	8/80	8/80	1–2
Pec dec	Chest	8/75	8/80	8/80	1–2
BB narrow grip bench presses	Chest	8/75	8/80	8/80	1–2
Wide gr. pullups	Back	12	14	16	1–3
Seated cable rowing	Back	8/75	8/80	8/85	1–2
DB seated overhead presses	Shoulder	8/65	8/75	8/80	1–2
DB shrugs	Trapezius	8/80	8/85	8/90	1–2
DB curls	Biceps	8/70	8/75	8/80	1–2
Tricep pressdowns	Triceps	8/70	8/75	8/80	1–2
Incline situps	Abdominals	20	25	30	1–2

Phase III

Exercise	Muscle Group	Repetitions & Resistance Level			Rest between Sets (minutes)
		Set 1	Set 2	Set 3	
Leg presses	Quadriceps, hamstrings	8/80	6/85	6/90	1–3
Leg curls	Hamstrings	8/70	8/80	6/85	1–2
DB calf raises	Calves	25/70	25/75	25/80	1–2
DB bench presses	Chest	8/80	6/85	6/90	1–2
Supine lat raises	Chest	8/70	6/80	6/80	1–2
Wide grip pullups	Back	13	15	17	1–2
DB rows	Back	8/75	6/85	6/85	1–2
BB seated overhead presses	Shoulders	8/75	6/85	6/90	1–2
Cable curls	Biceps	8/80	6/82	6/85	1–2
Weighted dips	Triceps	10/20 lb.	10/25 lb.	10/30 lb.	1–2
Tricep pressdowns	Triceps	8/80	6/85	6/90	1–2
Incline situps	Abdominals	15/5 lb.	15/10 lb.	15/15 lb	1–2
Leg raises	Abdominals, Hip	50	50	50	2

I hope that all of these programs will produce the most satisfying of results. Good lifting!

CHAPTER SEVEN

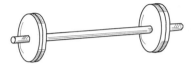

Weight Training Exercises

*I*n this chapter, strength training exercises are pictured and explained. They are organized by the muscle group or body part primarily affected. The muscles that cause the movement to occur when doing a particular exercise are referred to as *prime movers* or the *target musculature*. Some exercises require many muscle groups to function as prime movers (e.g., the clean).

Sometimes in weight training there is a tendency to think of an exercise as affecting only one muscle group (the prime mover group) when in reality most exercises cause a response in a number of other muscle groups as well. Indeed, a number of our muscles have no prime moving function at all. Their sole purpose is to stabilize joints. We refer to these muscles as *synergists*. When we set out to improve our muscular fitness or strength, strengthening these synergists is as important as strengthening prime movers.

SOME OBSERVATIONS ON WEIGHT TRAINING MACHINES

Over the past several years manufacturers of weight training equipment have made machines that *isolate* muscle groups. The kind of prime mover isolation caused by machines with weight stacks, handles, and foot pedals that all move on paths determined by glide posts or pivot points that allow no lateral movement can be good for the human body when a particular muscle group has been injured and is going through a recovery process. However, these isolation machines that thoroughly challenge the prime movers, challenge the stabilizing muscles to a lesser degree. How much less is difficult to say. Electromyographic studies simply show less muscle activity among the synergistic muscles during exercise with machines than when doing similar exercises with free weights (1). If this is true, and our evidence supports this, using these machines could produce an imbalance in muscular strength—strong prime movers and less strong synergists, a condition that predisposes one to injury.

The opposite of isolation is generality or nonspecificity. The most extreme example of this type of strength training might be Milo wrestling with an animal as he tried to hoist it to his shoulders. Perhaps the most general type of strength training done today is single-limb or dumbbell exercise, wherein each limb must independently balance and lift the weight through the required range of motion. This type of lifting maximizes synergistic muscle activity.

Weight training machines have been manufactured for many reasons. Most machines are easy and convenient to use, and they are thought to be safer than free weights. However, two of the worst injuries I have ever seen in a weight room were caused by machines. A falling weight stack smashed someone's hand and a person's shins were raked when his feet slipped off the leg-press foot pedals. Machines that use air or hydraulic pistons for resistance are safer than those that use weight stacks. Doctors and physical therapists like the isokinetic machines they use to rehabilitate patients. (See Chapter Two for a discussion of isokinetic machines.) Machines have been manufactured because they are the convenient and easily organized, allowing workouts to be completed simply by completing a circuit of machines. Another primary reason for making machines has been to try to put our bodies in positions that work muscle groups better or differently than can be done using free weights. But perhaps the major reason for machines in weight training is to earn money for the manufacturer.

Machines appeal to us all. When we walk into a weight room where the machines gleam and loom in all their apparent high-tech complexity, we are automatically impressed. This is the modern age of fitness. We expect something reflecting our state of technology, and the manufacturers are only too willing to provide such things for us—at a cost. Imagine going from a room equipped with computerized resistance equipment into a weight room with only free weights in evidence. The average person would consider the free-weight room antiquated! It is my judgement that a well-conceived weight training program using free weights cannot be improved on—unless perhaps Milo's technique is included in the workout.

BIOMECHANICAL DESCRIPTIONS OF CERTAIN BODY MOVEMENTS

In describing the exercises that follow I may use some terminology unfamiliar to you. This terminology is defined here for your reference.

Concentric contraction: The phase of a muscle contraction in which the prime movers or target musculature shorten(s). Muscle shortening can cause either flexion or extension at a joint (see below for definitions of flexion and extension).

Eccentric contraction: The phase of a muscle contraction in which the prime movers or target musculature lengthen(s). Such lengthening can result in either flexion or extension at a joint.

Flexion: The act of causing the angle between body parts (arms, fingers, or legs) to become smaller by contracting certain muscles. Whenever a muscle shortens (concentric contraction), another muscle on the opposite side of the joint lengthens (eccentric contraction). For example, when the biceps contract (elbow flexion), the forearm moves closer to the upper arm, and the triceps lengthen.

Plantar flexion is best understood by standing on your feet and then rising up on your toes (balls of your feet). In this movement the *heel* moves closer to the lower leg.

Dorsi flexion is the opposite of plantar flexion, raising the front part of your foot toward the lower leg, which brings the *forefoot* closer to the lower leg.

Extension: The act of causing the angle between body parts to become larger by contracting certain muscles. For example, when the quadriceps contract to cause *knee extension,* the lower leg moves farther from the upper leg.

Abduction: The act of moving a body part *laterally away* from the midline of the body (e.g., moving the arms away from the sides to a position parallel to the surface on which you are standing).

Adduction: The act of moving a body part *laterally toward* the midline of the body (e.g., moving the arms from a position directly out from the shoulders to the sides).

Smooth movement: This suggests that a movement should be done without jerkiness. Some exercises require explosive force (e.g., the clean), but this does not suggest jerkiness. Some exercises should be done at a faster cadence than others but still in a smooth manner. When powerlifters attempt extremely heavy lifts a phenomenon known as *synchronization* (simultaneous firing of many motor units) may result.

This produces a jerkiness that certainly is not smooth. This phenomenon is the body's response to extreme strength demands.

Pronation and supination: Prone means face down, and supine means face up. These terms are also used to define hand positions when gripping a bar. Pronated means a grip with the palm facing down or toward the body; supinated means a grip with the palm facing up or away from the body.

EXERCISES FOR THE LEG AND HIP

Lower Leg (Calf)

When you point your toe or stand on your toes the gastrocnemius and soleus muscles contract. This action is *plantar flexion,* in the terminology of human movement. The opposite motion, raising the forefoot by contracting the anterior tibialis, is known as *dorsiflexion.* These two terms are integral to this section.

For each of the calf exercises do one set with the feet parallel, one set with the heels turned in, and one set with the heels turned out. Doing so thoroughly exercises the calf muscles.

1. **Dumbbell Calf Raises (Figure 7–1)**
    Target musculature: Gastrocnemius, Soleus
    Description: Find a raised area in the weight room, preferably the edge of a platform, and hold on to a squat rack or other upright close by for stability. Grasp a dumbbell in the hand of the same side as the leg you wish to exercise. Put the ball of the exercising foot on the edge of the platform and move from complete plantar flexion to complete dorsiflexion. Brace the foot of the nonexercising leg on the back of the exercising leg.

2. **Barbell Calf Raises (Figure 7–2)**
    Target musculature: Gastrocnemius, Soleus
    Description: With a barbell across the shoulders, stand with the balls of both feet on the edge of a platform or other foot block. Carefully lower your body until your feet are completely dorsiflexed, then raise up until the feet are fully plantarflexed (standing high on the balls of the feet). This exercise requires precise balancing.

3. **Seated Heel Raises with Barbell (Figure 7–3)**
    Target musculature: Gastrocnemius, Soleus
    Description: Find a bench or stool tall enough so that when you sit on it your thighs are parallel with the floor. Place a block 2 or 3 inches thick under the balls of your feet, but keep your lower leg vertical. Place a pad

Figure 7–1
Dumbbell calf
raises

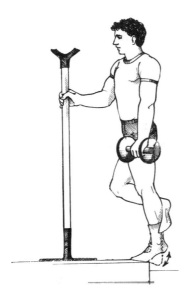

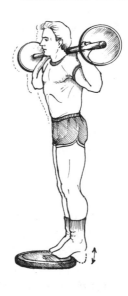

Figure 7–2
Barbell calf raises

across your thighs. Then, with the assistance of a training partner, position a barbell on the pad just above your knees. Hold the bar in place as you completely dorsiflex and plantarflex your ankles.

4. Toe Presses (Figure 7–4)

Target musculature: Gastrocnemius, Soleus

Description: This exercise is done on the leg press station of a variety of weight stack-type machines. Adjust the seat so the weight stack only rises 8 to 10 inches when your legs are fully extended. In this extended position, carefully adjust your feet until the balls of your feet are positioned on the edge of the foot pedals. *Make sure that the balls of your feet are securely on the foot pedals so there is no chance they might slip off while doing the exercise.* Plantarflex and dorsiflex fully to assure exercise through the complete range of motion.

Figure 7–3
Seated heel
raises with barbell

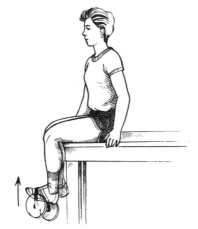

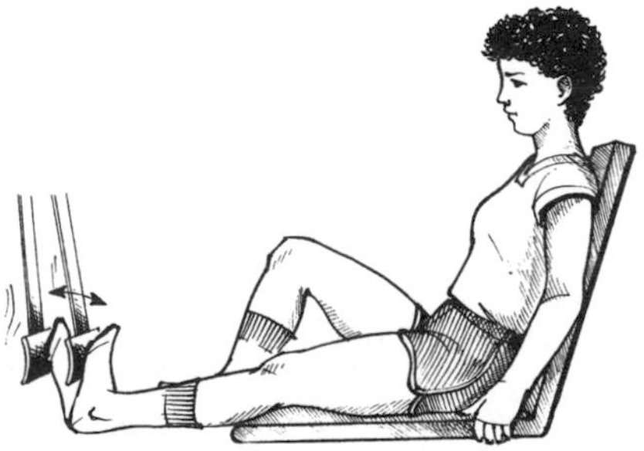

Figure 7–4
Toe presses

5. **Toe Raises (Figure 7–5)**

Target musculature: Anterior tibialis

Description: For this exercise you need a high bench or table, a short rope, and a free-weight plate. Sit with your lower legs hanging over the end of the table. Tie the rope through a weight with enough slack to loop the rope over the fore part of your foot. Dorsiflex and plantarflex your foot through the full range. Hold your toes up to keep the rope from slipping off the foot during the plantar flexion phase.

Upper Leg (Thigh) and Hip

1. **Squats (Figure 7–6)**

Target musculature: Quadriceps, Hamstrings, Gluteus maximus

Description: The squat is a great exercise that works muscles across many joints of the body. When beginning the exercise, it is important to lift *light* weight until you become competent and your legs and back adjust to this new stress.

With the bar on a weight rack, position yourself so that the bar is centered on your shoulders. Lift the bar entirely clear of the rack and *carefully* back out of the rack far enough that the natural forward bend when squatting does not result in the bar hitting the rack. This forward bend should not be excessive. (The primary reason for backing out of the rack is to enable you to see the rack when you replace the bar at the end of the set)

When you set up for the squat your feet should be about shoulder width apart, with the feet turned out slightly. When lowering the body in a squat keep the knees over the toes. Determining the proper depth to lower your body is certainly important. I recommend that you carefully *in a controlled movement,* drop to a position where the lower part of your thighs (ham-

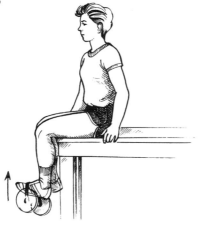

Figure 7–5
Toe raises

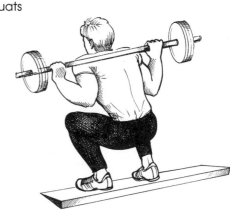

Figure 7–6
Squats

strings) are roughly parallel with the floor. *Remember to keep the back straight and your head up* as you drop into this position. This will give the thighs and hips a good stretch and assure strength development through a full range of motion without excessively stressing the knee joint.

2. Lunges (Figure 7–7)

Target musculature: Quadriceps, Hamstrings, Gluteus maximus, Calves

Description: Position a properly weighted barbell on your shoulders. Lift the barbell off the squat rack and step back away from the rack. After assuming a parallel stance, take a long step forward and allow your *forward* leg to bend at the knee until the thigh is parallel with the floor. The rear leg is kept almost straight, which puts a good stretch on the hip flexor muscles that cross in front of the hip joint. After achieving this position, return to a parallel stance, switch legs, and do the same movement with the other leg forward.

3. Power Clean (Figure 7–8)

Target musculature: Quadriceps, Hamstrings, Calves, Gluteus maximus, Erector spinae, Trapezius

Description: Position your feet shoulder width apart in front of the bar. Bending at the hip, knee, and ankle joints, squat down and grasp the bar in a pronated grip. Keeping the back straight, the arms extended, and the bar close to your body, lift the weight from the floor with your legs. As the bar rises just past the knees, thrust the shoulders strongly upward at the same time as you drive the hips forward and up. Rise up on your toes and pull with the trapezius muscles to continue the upward movement of the bar until the bar can be "racked" in a shoulder-height position.

Figure 7–7
Lunges

Figure 7–8
Power cleans

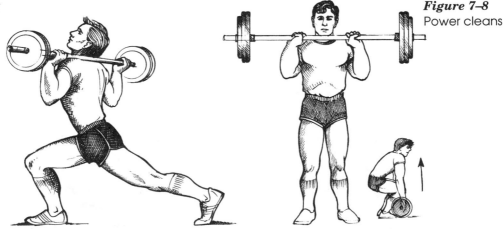

Figure 7–9
Leg Presses

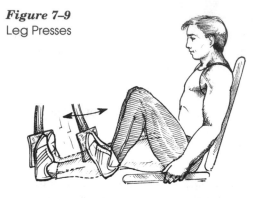

Figure 7–10
Hip sleds

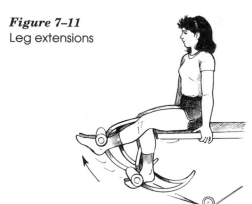

Figure 7–11
Leg extensions

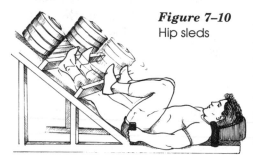

Figure 7–12
Leg curls

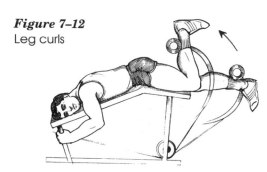

4. Leg Presses (Figure 7–9)

Target musculature: Quadriceps, Hamstrings, Gluteus maximus

Description: Many manufacturers have built machines that include leg press stations. These machines normally consist of an adjustable seat, foot pedals attached to a lever system, and an adjustable weight stack at the end of the lever system.

A major concern of the exerciser is how close to position the seat to the foot pedals. Too close puts the body in a poor position for movement—too far away does not require the muscles to go through a full range of movement. Experiment to find the correct position. Grip the hand-holds on the sides of the seat while extending the legs; press the weight to full extension; and then in a controlled but not overly slow manner return the weight to the starting position.

5. Hip Sleds (Figure 7–10)

Target musculature: Quadriceps, Hamstrings, Gluteus Maximus

Description: Hip sleds can be used either as leg press machines, by lying on your back pushing with the legs, or as blocking machines, by standing and driving the weight with the shoulders.

Most machines have two adjustable sites: one on the portion that holds the weight and the other where the back is positioned (in the case of the leg press), or where the feet are positioned (in the blocking movement). When doing either the leg press or the blocking move adjust the machine so you get a good stretch of the working muscles at the completion of the eccentric phase. Caution: When doing the blocking movement, do not hyperextend the hips/lower back during the concentric phase of the exercise.

6. Leg Extension (Figure 7–11)

Target musculature: Quadriceps

Description: Leg extension machines consist of a seat, a lifting lever (usually adjustable) with padded laterals for the lower legs, and a cable system running from the lifting lever to a weight stack.

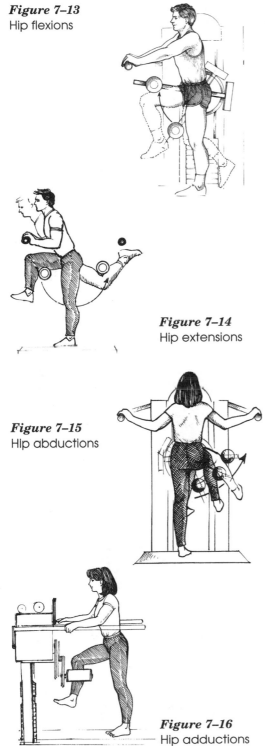

Figure 7–13
Hip flexions

Figure 7–14
Hip extensions

Figure 7–15
Hip abductions

Figure 7–16
Hip adductions

Sit comfortably in the seat, place your legs behind the padded laterals and completely extend the lower leg(s). Return the weight smoothly to the start position. Make the movement crisp and rhythmic throughout the set.

7. Leg Curls (Figure 7–12)

Target musculature: Hamstrings

Description: There are three types of leg curl machines: (1) flat benches, (2) benches with shallow V shapes, and (3) machines for doing leg curls in a standing position. All of these machines use a lever system (usually adjustable in length) with padded laterals and a cable system attached to a weight stack. In my opinion, the most comfortable are those with moderate "V-ing" of the bench.

Lie face down on the bench and hook your legs under the padded laterals. Adjust the lever so your knee cap is beyond the bench and the padded laterals are comfortably above your heels. Maintain this position throughout the entire range of movement.

8. Multi-Hip Machines

Target musculature: Rectus femoris, Hamstrings, Gluteus maximus, Leg abductors, Leg adductors.

Description: Multi hip machines have been created primarily in response to the requests of women who want more exercises to thoroughly work the thigh and hip areas. The machines consist of an adjustable length lever which can be set at different positions on a circular axis. The lever has a padded lateral. The circular axis is further attached to a weight stack via a cable system. Bars to hold for maintaining balance while exercising are strategically positioned on the machines. The four movements possible on these machines are hip flexions (Figure 7–13), hip extensions (Figure 7–14), hip abductions (Figure 7–15), and hip adductions (Figure 7–16). Positioning the padded lateral to get the full range of resistance is of major importance. When doing adduction and abduction, it is also important that the padded lateral does not hit the nonexercising leg.

EXERCISES FOR THE ABDOMINAL AND WAIST AREAS

A word about abdominal exercise for your information. When doing a situp (trunk flexion & hip flexion), the prime movers are the rectus abdominus and the hip flexors. The rectus abdominus contracts or shortens to bring the sternum (rib cage) as close to the pubic bone as possible. Once this is accomplished the rectus abdominus does not shorten further. This range of motion for trunk flexion is completed during the first few degrees of the situp movement. After that, the hip flexors move the torso while the abdominal muscles maintain a static contraction. The abdominal muscles work throughout the full range but primarily in a static state. *Twisting* abdominal exercies are necessary to exercise the oblique and transverse muscles of the midsection.

Reducing the amount of fat around our midsections is something many of us hope for. Abdominal exercise is good for tightening up sagging muscles, but trying to spot-reduce by exercising certain areas of the body has not been proven to be effective.

1.   Bent Knee Situp (Figure 7–17)

Target musculature: Primarily rectus abdominus (all abdominals), Hip flexors (Rectus femoris, Ilio psoas, Pectineus)

Description: This basic exercise is the standard one for the midsection. The exerciser should lie flat on his or her back, knees bent at least 90 degrees, with hands behind the neck, alongside the head, or placed high on the chest. (The higher the hands, the more stress on the working muscles.) Hooking your feet under a bar is a common technique, but doing so probably puts more stress on the hip flexors than on the abdominal

Figure 7–17
Bent knee situps

Figure 7–18
Seated bar twists

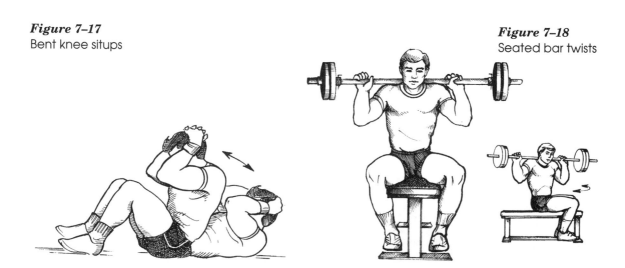

muscle. You should curl up, assuring that the head rises first, then the chest. Try to keep the lower back on the floor until the chest is well off. This sequence of movement assures proper abdominal exercise. As you become stronger, resistance can be increased by lying head down on an incline board or by holding a weight on the chest.

2. **Seated Bar Twists (Figure 7–18)**

    Target musculature: Oblique muscles of the abdomen

    Description: For this exercise you will need a bench that can be straddled and a light, straight bar. Straddle the bench, sit down, place the bar across the shoulders behind the neck. Hands should be out on the bar, away from the shoulders. (The bar can be a broom handle or other light bar.) Lock your legs so there is no turning of the hips. Twist completely to the left then return to the start position, then twist completely to the right and back to the start position. The cadence should be crisp, neither purposely slow nor violently fast. This exercise can be done standing, but it is easier to lock the hips while sitting. Work up to 100 repetitions.

3. **Twisting Situps (Figure 7–19)**

    Target musculature: Rectus abdominus and abdominal obliques

    Description: Start flat on your back on an exercise mat or a thick carpet, with your knees bent at least 90 degrees, feet flat on the floor, and hands behind your head. By contracting the abdominal muscles, first bring your head, then your chest off the floor, twisting as you rise so that you can touch one elbow to the opposite knee. Return to the starting position, then repeat, touching the opposite elbow to the other knee.

4. **Crunch Situps (Figure 7–20)**

    Target musculature: Abdominals

    Description: Lying with your back and hips flat on an exercise mat, place your lower legs over a bench. Adjust your body so that your thighs are vertical. Place your hands behind your head then contract your abdominal muscles and bring your elbows forward until they make contact

Figure 7–19
Twisting situps

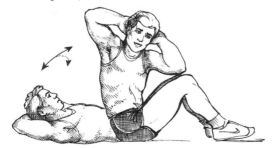

Figure 7–20
Crunch situps

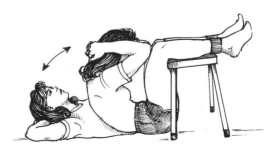

with your thighs. Return to the starting position and repeat. (This exercise quite effectively minimizes use of the hip flexors.)

5. **Leg Raises and Kneeups (Figure 7–21)**
   Target musculature: Hip flexors and lower abdominal muscles
   Description: You can do leg raises and knee up exercises lying on your back, sitting on the edge of a high bench, hanging, or supporting yourself on your elbows in an erect position. You can also increase the stress on the working muscles by straightening the leg and/or moving to a more erect body position. The kneeup exercise is known as *hip flexion* in human movement. The prime moving muscles are the hip flexors. However, there is a static contraction of the lower fibers of the rectus abdominus associated with this exercise. Most weight trainers of some experience will attest to the beneficial effects of leg raises or kneeups for tightening up the lower abdomen. When in position, rhythmically lift the knees as high as possible and then return them to the starting position. (Lying kneeups are often used by beginning exercisers who are too weak to do situps.)

6. **Side Bends (Figure 7–22)**
   Target musculature: Lateral flexors, Erector spinae, Abdominals
   Description: This exercise will firm waist, hips, and abdominal muscles. Stand tall with a dumbbell hanging in one hand. Bend carefully to the side with the dumbbell until you feel a stretch of the opposite side. Return crisply to an upright position.

7. **Roman Chair Abdominal Work (Figure 7–23)**
   Target musculature: Hip flexors and abdominal muscles
   Description: This exercise should be used only by the very well-conditioned exerciser; the stress placed on the lower back and hip flexors can be

Figure 7–21
Leg raises and
knee ups

Figure 7–22
Side Bends

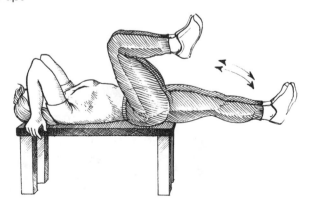

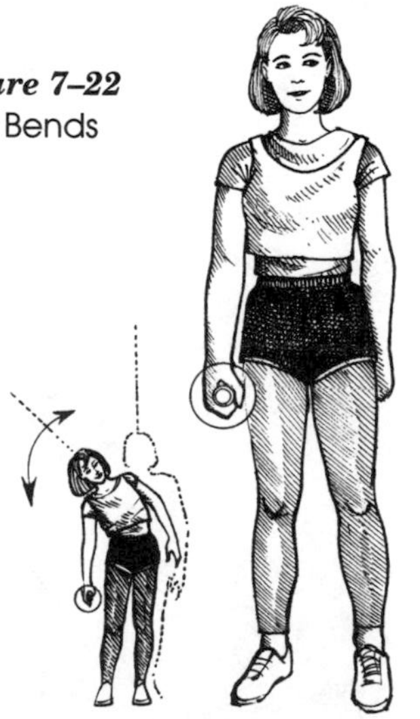

extreme. When the exerciser's shoulders drop below the level of the buttocks, the abdominals are placed on stretch, thus working them through a more complete range than most other abdominal exercises. The exercise may be performed over a bench or on an apparatus designed especially for it. Sit across a bench with feet stabilized. Carefully lower your torso to the rear until you feel a comfortable stretch of the abdominals. *Do not drop to a position that causes pain in the lower back.* Raise the torso to an upright position by contracting the hip flexors and abdominal muscles.

EXERCISES FOR THE CHEST

1. **Bench Press (Figure 7–24)**

    Target musculature: Pectoralis major, Anterior deltoid, Triceps

    Description: When you lift free weights you should have a spotter. Start flat on your back. Place your hands a little wider than shoulder width on the bar resting on the rack above your neck. When ready, have your spotter assist you in lifting the bar off the rack to arm's length above your chest. When you have the bar fully under control, carefully lower the bar to your chest until it touches just below the breast line, then drive the bar back up to the arms-extended position.

    The grip position on the bar can be moved from narrow (4-6 in. between the thumbs) to wide (up to 40 in. between thumbs) to affect different fibers of the pectoralis major. The position the bar touches on the body can also be moved for different muscular stress. This position can vary from just below the breast line to as high as the neck. Bench presses can be done with either a barbell or dumbbells.

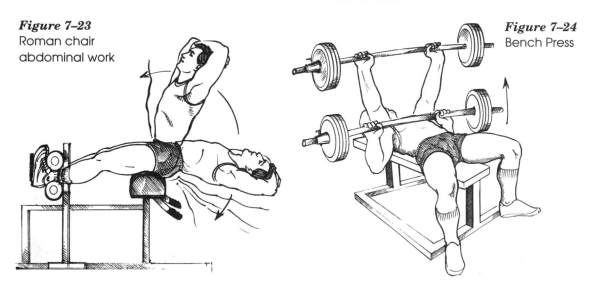

Figure 7–23
Roman chair abdominal work

Figure 7–24
Bench Press

2. **Incline Bench Press (Figure 7–25)**

Target musculature: Pectoralis major, Anterior deltoid, Triceps

Description: Incline benches are of two types: those on which you lie, which have foot pedals for stability, and those on which you sit. The angle the benches are inclined is usually around 45 degrees. The incline bench press can be done with either dumbbells or a barbell. Some incline benches are built with racks for barbells.

Take a position with your back solidly against the bench. Move the weight to full arm's extension above the chest (a spotter may be needed for this), then lower them down to a position near the clavicles (high on the chest), and then drive back up to full arm's extension.

3. **Bent Arm Pullovers (Figure 7–26)**

Target musculature: Pectoralis major, Latissimus dorsi, Triceps

Description: For this exercise you need a bench on which you lie on your back with your head hanging over the end. Lock your legs around the bench so your shoulders don't slip off. Have a spotter hand you the bar, which should then be placed high on your chest. Assuring that the bar clears your face, push it up and back, then let gravity pull it below your head as far as is comfortable. Allow as much stretch as is comfortable as the bar is lowered. Be certain to keep your elbows close to your head—do not allow them to flange out as the movement progresses. Once your arms are fully extended, bring the bar back up to a position high on the chest just below the shoulders.

4. **Supine Lateral Raises (Flies) (Figure 7–27)**

Target musculature: Anterior deltoid, Pectoralis major

Figure 7–25
Incline bench
press

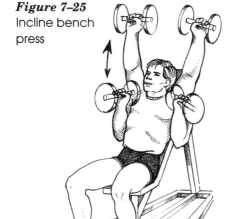

Figure 7–26
Bent arm
pullovers

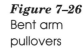

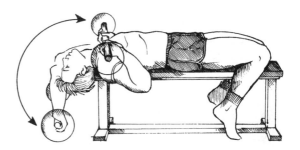

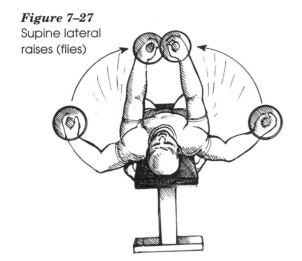

Figure 7-27
Supine lateral
raises (flies)

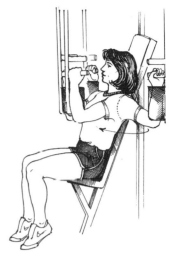

Figure 7-28
Pec Dec

Description: This exercise is done lying on your back with both arms extended laterally away from the body. A dumbbell is held in each hand. The exercise can be done with your arms completely straight (not recommended except with very light weight) or with varying degrees of bend at the elbow. Plant your feet flat on the floor for good balance and move the weights from a comfortably stretched, low position until they gently touch above the chest. For best results, turn your hands so the palms face each other as they come together above the chest.

5. **Pec Dec (Figure 7-28)**

   Target musculature: Pectoralis major

   Description: Sit down on the seat of the pec dec machine. With your elbows bent 90 degrees, raise your arms laterally and place them behind the pads on each side of you. Your lower arms should be essentially vertical behind the pads. Pull the pads together in front of you, then let them return to the starting position.

EXERCISES FOR THE BACK

Lower Back

1. **Deadlift & Straight Leg Deadlift (Figure 7-29)**

   Target musculature: Erector spinae, Gluteus maximus, Quadriceps, Hamstrings

   Description: Doing deadlifts exercises many of the major moving muscles of the body, but the major focus of the exercise is on the lower back. With the bar on a lifting platform, take a stance with your feet shoulder width apart and the bar very close to your shin bones. Bending your knees and keeping your back quite straight, lower your body until you can grasp the bar, with one hand pronated and the other supinated. The hands should be positioned outside of the lower legs. With the head up and the back straight, extend the knee and hip joints to lift the bar from the platform. As the bar passes the knees your back should straighten, bringing the torso into an erect position, with the bar hanging at arm's length. Lowering the bar (eccentric phase) for another repetition is the opposite movement.

A variation of the true deadlift is the straight leg deadlift. The difference is simply that the knees are not allowed to bend during the movement, thus placing all of the resistance on the lower back and the gluteal muscles of the hip. This exercise concentrates great stress in the lower back; therefore your should use only light weight when beginning.

2. Good Morning Exercise (Figure 7–30)

Target musculature: Erector spinae, Gluteus maximus, Hamstrings

Description: This exercise gets its name from a former time, when it was customary to bow as you wished someone good morning. It can be somewhat uncomfortable, as the bar presses into the spine and muscles of the shoulders and posterior neck. Proper padding helps.

Set up the bar on a squat rack then pad your shoulders—lightly, so you don't lose the feel of the bar. Balance the bar on your shoulders and back away from the rack. Keeping the bar as low on your shoulders as is comfortable, bend forward as if you were doing a bow. Keeping the back relatively flat places the major stress on the hamstrings and gluteus; letting the back round somewhat places more stress on the erector spinae of the lower back.

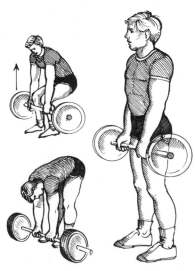

Figure 7–29
Deadlift and straight leg deadlift

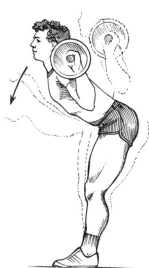

Figure 7–30
Good morning exercise

3. Back Hyperextensions (Figure 7–31)

Target musculature: Erector spinae, Gluteus maximus, Hamstrings

Description: This exercise can be performed over any high table or bench that allows the torso to hang down without the head touching the floor. Benches with feet-locking mechanisms make doing this exercise quite convenient. If you don't have this type of bench you will need a strap to hold your legs in place, or a partner to do so.

With your hips comfortably placed on the padded edge of the bench or table, put your hands behind your head and lower your torso until it is essentially vertical. (A major fault when doing this exercise is not dropping into a full vertical position.) Rise up until your back breaks parallel with the floor. Rising up to a position where your chest is high above your buttocks may put a strain on the lower back. It is therefore recommended that the back be brought up only to a position slightly above parallel with the floor. The exercise should be done in a rhythmic, flowing manner, not fast or slow.

Middle and Upper Back

1. Bent-Over Rowing (Figure 7–32)

Target musculature: Latissimus dorsi, Rhomboids, Posterior deltoid, Trapezius, Biceps

Description: This lift is often done with a bar between the legs, weighted on only one end; or by standing on blocks to allow greater stretch of the working muscles. Use caution when beginning this exercise: you can strain the lower back if you try to lift too much weight.

Stand as you would when beginning a clean, the bar directly above your toes, feet shoulder-width apart. Bend the knees and hips until you can take a good pronated grip of the bar, lift the hips slightly until the bar

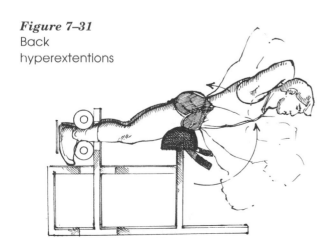

Figure 7–31
Back
hyperextentions

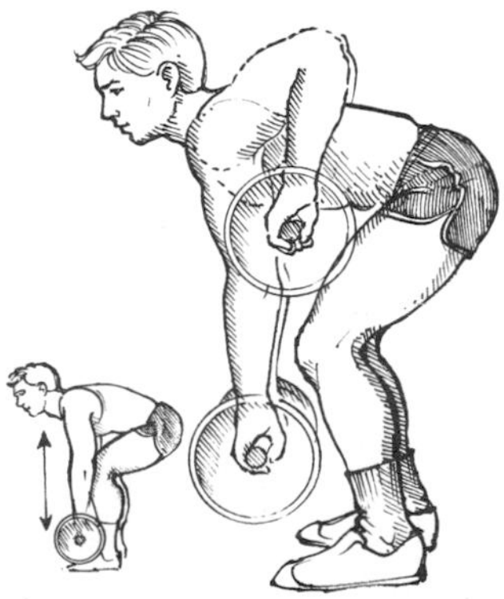

Figure 7–32
Bent-over rowing

clears the floor, then staying in the bent-over position, bring the bar up to your chest by contracting the muscles across your back and flexing your elbows.

2.   Pullups or Chinups (Figure 7–33)

Target musculature: Latissimus dorsi, Biceps, Brachioradialis
Description: With the hands pronated, the brachioradialis (muscle below the elbow on the outside of the arm) is worked considerably more than with the hands supinated. Either a pronated or supinated grip allows a good workout of the latissimus dorsi muscle, but the biceps are worked more with the supinated grip. Wide, pronated-grip pullups, where your head comes in front of the bar, are most specific to the latissimus dorsi muscle.

Start in a position hanging from a bar, with feet clear of the floor. Pull your body up until your chin is above the bar. Lower yourself, under control, back to the starting position.

3.   One-Arm Dumbbell Rowing (Figure 7–34)

Target musculature: Latissimus dorsi, Biceps
Description: With a dumbbell in your right hand stand next to a bench so that it is on your left side. Place your left lower leg on the bench and bend at the waist until your left hand is supporting part of your weight on the bench. Your back should be essentially parallel with the floor. With your exercising arm at full extension, pull the weight up to your torso, and then lower it back carefully, under control to full extension.

4.   Reverse Flies (Figure 7–35)

Target musculature: Posterior deltoids, Rhomboids, Trapezius

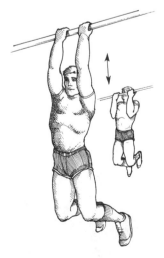

Figure 7–33
Pullups or
chinups

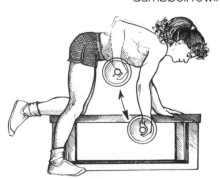

Figure 7–34
One-arm
dumbbell rowing

Description: With a dumbbell in each hand, bend forward, keeping your back relatively flat, until your back is at about a 30-degree angle with the floor. Bend your arms to about a 90-degree angle, and with palms facing each other, lift the weights out laterally and up as high as possible. Control the weights as you return them to the starting position.

5. Wide-Grip Lat Pulldowns (Figure 7–36)

Target musculature: Latissimus dorsi, Biceps, Brachioradialis

Description: This exercise is one of the most popular in any weight room. The lat pulldown is the same as the wide-grip pullup except that the resistance is now provided by a machine. Keeping your back vertical, pull the bar down behind your neck until it touches your shoulders. Then, in a controlled manner, allow the weight to return to a full arms-extended position. When the resistance you can use approximates your body weight, you will need some means of holding your body down. Training partners can hold you down by applying pressure to your shoulders. Bars can be placed across your calves, if you kneel, or across your thighs if you sit down.

6. Reverse-Grip Lat Pulldowns (Figure 7–37)

Target musculature: Latimissus dorsi, Biceps

Description: Grasp the lat pulldown bar with a supinated grip, hands not more than 12 inches apart. Kneel or sit down (use a training partner or weight to hold you down if necessary) and, pulling with your arms, draw the bar down until it comes well below the chin, then let the bar return to the starting position, using control.

7. Seated Cable Rowing (Figure 7–38)

Target musculature: Latissimus dorsi, Posterior deltoid, Rhomboids, Biceps

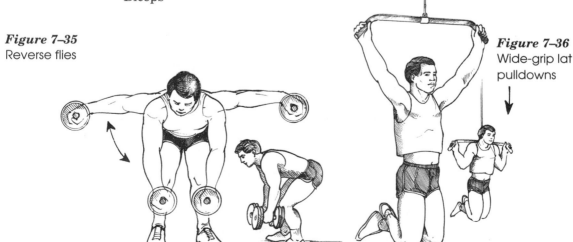

Figure 7–35
Reverse flies

Figure 7–36
Wide-grip lat
pulldowns
↓

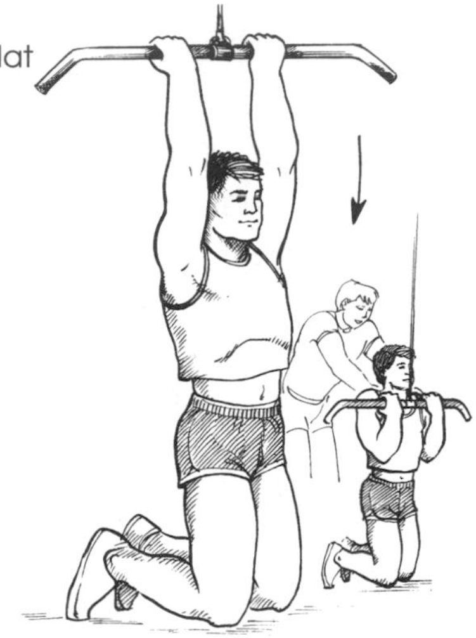

Figure 7–37
Reverse-grip lat
pulldowns

Figure 7–38
Seated cable
rowing

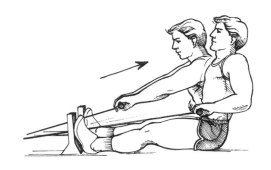

Description: Sit with your legs fully extended in front of a low lat pull machine. Your feet may need to be blocked some distance in front of the machine to allow for a complete range of motion. Reach forward and grasp the bar or handle attached to the cable, then bring your torso to an upright position and keep it there throughout the exercise. With your torso erect, extend your arms fully, then pull them in until the bar touches your abdomen about naval height. Do not sway as you do the repetitions.

EXERCISES FOR THE SHOULDERS

Although many muscles surround and give strength and movement to the shoulder, in the world of strength training shoulder has come to mean primarily the deltoid muscle, which sits atop the shoulders. This large muscle has an anterior or frontal head, a superior or middle head, and a posterior head. The primary action of the deltoid is to move our arms laterally away from our bodies (shoulder abduction), but the anterior head is very active in horizontal shoulder flexion (bringing the arm closer to the torso on a horizontal plane), and the posterior head causes horizontal shoulder extension (moving the arm horizontally away from our front toward our back.

1.   **The Overhead Press (Figure 7–39)**
     Target musculature: Deltoid (anterior and middle heads), Triceps
     Description: This exercise can be done either standing or sitting, with either a barbell or dumbbells. Bring the bar to a position parallel with the shoulders, with hands in a pronated grip positioned just outside

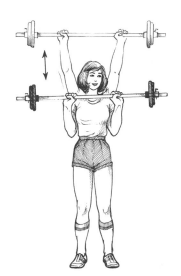

Figure 7–39
Overhead press

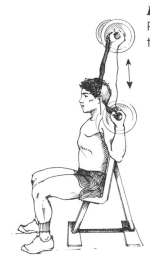

Figure 7–40
Press behind
the neck

the shoulders. From there, push the bar overhead until the arms are fully extended. Lower the bar carefully back to the starting position.

2. **Press behind the Neck (Figure 7–40)**

   Target musculature: Deltoid (anterior and middle heads), Triceps
   Description: This exercise is sometimes referred to as the *shoulder press*. The only difference between this exercise and the overhead press is that the bar is started from a position resting on the shoulders behind the neck. More specificity can be achieved by sitting in a back-supported position.

3. **Upright Rowing (Figure 7–41)**

   Target musculature: Deltoid (all heads), Biceps, Trapezius
   Description: Grasp a bar with a pronated grip, placing your index fingers 4 to 6 inches apart. Stand erect, with the bar hanging at arm's length and feet shoulder-width apart. Contracting the deltoid and bicep muscles,

Figure 7–41
Upright
rowing

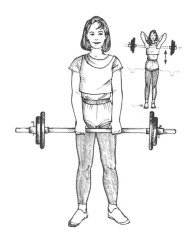

lift the bar to a position just below your chin while keeping the elbows as high as possible. Carefully lower the bar back to the starting position. Do not swing the bar or bend forward.

4. **Dumbbell Standing Lateral Raise (Figure 7–42)**

   Target musculature: Deltoid, Trapezius

   Description: This exercise can be done keeping the body erect and the arms straight, stopping the dumbbells at the sides of the hips, or in the more common position of a slight forward bend of the hips and somewhat bent elbows to allow the weights to pass in front of the body in the starting position.

   Start in a standing position, with a dumbbell in each hand, palms facing each other weights in front of your body below belt height, slightly bent forward at the waist. Lift the weights outward and upward until they reach a position above your shoulders. *Keep your palms down to keep stress on the entire deltoid.* As the weights clear your hips, come to an erect position. As you control the return of the weight to the starting position, bend slightly forward so the weight can pass in front of the hips.

5. **Front Raises (Figure 7–43)**

   Target musculature: Deltoid (anterior and middle heads)

   Description: Stand with a dumbbell in each hand. Keeping the arms relatively straight, raise your arms, together or alternately, out in front of you until your hand rises above your shoulder. Keep the palm facing the floor as the weight is raised. Return the weight to the starting position under control.

Figure 7–42
Dumbbell standing lateral raise

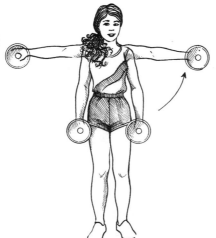

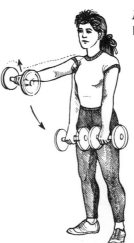

Figure 7–43
Front raises

EXERCISES FOR THE ARM

Upper Arm and Elbow Flexors

Arm curls (elbow flexion) can be done with barbells, dumbbells, or any of a significant variety of machines. Curls with dumbbells can be done sitting or standing. Curls are all, with one exception, done with a supinated grip. Supinated means a grip wherein the palms face up, to the front, or away from the body. The one exception is *reverse curls*. The name implies a position opposite or the reverse of that which is normal; hence reverse curls are done with a pronated grip.

1. **Arm Curls (Figure 7–44)**
    Target musculature: Biceps, Brachialis
    Description: Using a supinated grip, grip a bar and come to a standing position, with the bar hanging at full arm's extension in front of your body. The bar can be a straight bar, or what is known as an *E Z curl bar*, which is angled to put the biceps in a stronger position than would be the case with a straight bar. Without swinging or swaying, curl the bar to a position just in front of your shoulders, then lower the bar under control back to the starting position. When doing the curl with dumbbells it is important to keep the hand *supinated* so the palms face generally upward. Allowing the palms to twist so they face each other (thumbs up) puts a major portion of the stress of the movement on the brachioradialis muscle, not on the biceps. This movement is referred to as a *hammer curl*. When doing dumbbell curls it is advantageous to alternate arms, as opposed to curling with both at the same time.

Figure 7–44
Arm curls

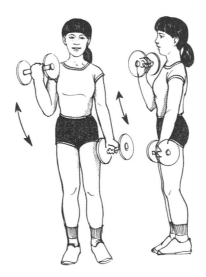

2.   **Seated Dumbbell Incline Curls (Figure 7–45)**

Target musculature: Biceps, Brachialis

Description: This exercise requires the use of a sitting-type incline bench. The primary purpose of this curl movement is to stretch the biceps more than is possible when doing other curl movements. Sit on the incline bench, and ensuring that your shoulders remain in contact, alternately curl the dumbbells until they reach shoulder height. Assure that the biceps get a maximal stretch as each arm is lowered.

3.   **Preacher Bench Curls (Figure 7–46)**

Target musculature: Biceps, Brachialis

Description: This exercise derives its name from the bench used in the exercise, which could be construed to look somewhat like the lectern used to hold notes when someone (a preacher) makes a presentation. The primary purpose of the bench is to immobilize the upper arms in an inclined position so that all the stress of the weight is moved by the prime movers.

Sit on the preacher bench and grasp the bar with a supinated grip. Keeping the elbows relatively close, contract your elbow flexors until your forearms are vertical. Lowering the weight under control is essential in this exercise because the bench often ends just below the elbows. Uncontrolled dropping of the weight could cause serious hyperextension of the elbows.

4.   **Cable Curls (Figure 7–47)**

Target musculature: Biceps, Brachialis

Description: Stand in front of the low lat pulley station. Grasp a bar attached to the cable. Standing erect, arms fully extended with no slack in

Figure 7–45
Seated dumb-
bell incline curls

Figure 7–46
Preacher bench
curls

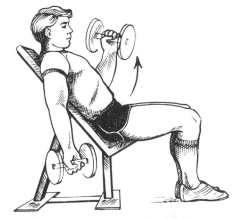

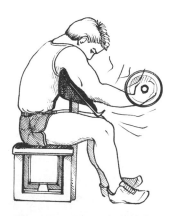

Figure 7–47
Cable curls

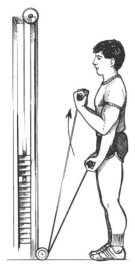

Figure 7–49
Reverse curls

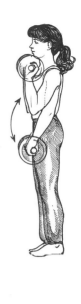

Figure 7–48
Machine curls

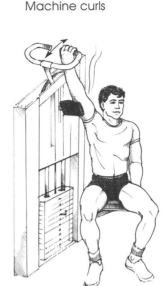

the cable, flex your biceps until the bar touches your chest. Return carefully to the starting position.

5. Machine Curls (Figure 7–48)

Target musculature: Biceps, Brachialis

Description: Many machines have chains, belts, and cables running from bars or other mechanisms to which you apply pressure over cams and/or pulleys to a weight stack. There are machines that use hydraulic resistance as well as machines that are computerized. The primary characteristic of all the machines is that they isolate the prime movers to a greater extent than does free-weight exercise. I tend not to favor exercises using machines. However, they are quite convenient and very popular.

6. Reverse Curls (Figure 7–49)

Target musculature: Brachioradialis, Biceps, Wrist extensors

Description: In a standing position grasp a bar with a *pronated* grip. By contracting the elbow flexors, and without swinging or swaying, bring the bar to a position just below the chin. Return the bar to the starting position under control.

Upper Arm and Elbow Extensors

1. **Seated Overhead Triceps Presses (French Presses)**
   (Figure 7–50)
   Target musculature: Triceps
   Description: When doing this exercise the weight is best distributed on both arms equally by using an E Z curl bar. If you choose not to use such a bar a dumbbell will suffice.

   Sit on a bench with some support at about the mid-point of your back. Sitting on a bench-press bench with your back resting on a bar on the rack is quite adequate. Lift the bar to full arm's extension overhead, keeping the elbows high and close to the head. Next allow the elbows to flex, lowering the weight behind the head. When the bar has reached a position well below the elbows, thrust the weight back to full arm's length above the head.

2. **Lying Triceps Presses (Figure 7–51)**
   Target musculature: Triceps
   Description: First, properly weight an E Z curl bar. Gripping the bar properly in a pronated grip, sit on the edge of a bench, then lie down, bringing the bar to a position arm's length above your head. From this position, allow the bar to descend, under control, to either just above the forehead (advanced lifter) or behind the head. Here, stop the downward motion, and thrust the bar back up overhead. Note that, dropping the bar

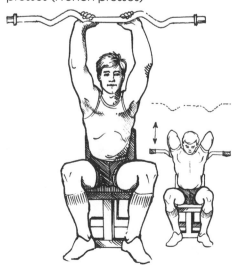

Figure 7–50
Seated overhead triceps
presses (French presses)

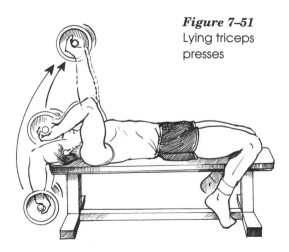

Figure 7–51
Lying triceps
presses

to the, *forehead* keeps the upper arm very stable, but dropping the bar behind the head requires that the upper arm move, producing somewhat of a undesirable swinging action.

3. Triceps Pressdowns (Figure 7–52)

Target musculature: Triceps

Description: This exercise requires the use of a lat pulldown machine. Take a relatively wide stance in front of the lat pulldown bar, grasp the bar in a pronated grip, and pull it down to a position approximately shoulder height. (Curved or triangular handles that put the triceps at the most advantageous position for applying force are usually available). Stop the bar momentarily at that position. Then, keeping the body from swaying, force the bar downward to complete arm's extension and then eccentrically allow it to return to shoulder-height position. Note that only when the set is complete should the bar move above the height of the shoulders.

4. Dips (Parallel Bar, Chair or Bench) (Figure 7–53)

Target musculature: Triceps

Description: Most exercise facilities have a set of bars that are intended to be used for dips. They are high enough that people can support their entire weight on the bars as they do the dip exercises. However, many people are not strong enough to safely do dips while lifting their entire body weight. For these people, chair or bench dips, where some of the weight is supported by the legs, is a much safer option.

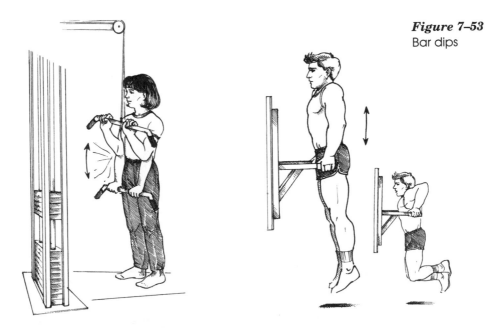

Figure 7–52
Triceps
pressdowns

Figure 7–53
Bar dips

When doing the bar dips, place your hands on the bars in a pronated grip, and with a jump of sufficient magnitude, mount the bars so that all your weight is taken by your arms. Keeping your lower legs flexed so that they do not touch the floor, lower your body until your upper arms are parallel with the floor. At that point, lift yourself back to an arms-extended position.

To do a chair or bench dip, stand with your back to a chair and, sit down, placing your hands behind you, palms down, over the edges of the chair. Be sure that the chair is stable. Lift your weight off the chair, move your buttocks in front of the chair, and extend your legs so only your heels are on the floor. Lower your weight until your buttocks are nearly touching the floor, then lift yourself back up to the arms-extended position.

5. Machine Triceps Work (Figure 7–54)

Target musculature: Triceps

Description: Many machines have chains, belts, and cables running from bars or other mechanisms to which you apply pressure, over cams and/or pulleys to a weight stack. And there are machines that use hydraulic resistance as well as machines that are computerized. The primary characteristic of all the machines is that they isolate the prime movers to a greater extent than does free weight exercise. I tend not to favor exercising using machines. However, they are quite convenient and very popular.

Figure 7–54
Nautilus tricep machine

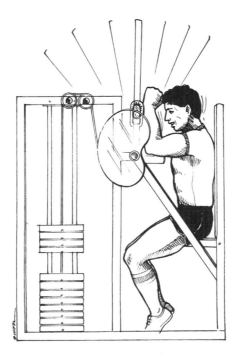

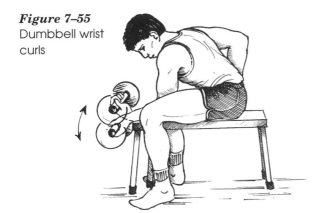

Figure 7–55
Dumbbell wrist
curls

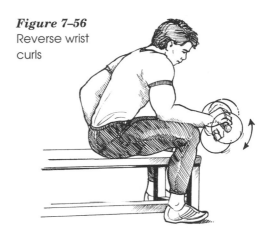

Figure 7–56
Reverse wrist
curls

EXERCISES FOR THE FOREARM

1. **Dumbbell Wrist Curls (Figure 7–55)**
    Target musculature: Wrist flexors
    Description: Grasp a dumbbell in the hand that is to be exercised first. Then sit down and place the back of the arm you wish to exercise on the thigh of the same side, palm up. The back of the wrist should be over the knee so that the hand, when allowed to open, is beyond the knee. In this position, extend the fingers (eccentric contraction) so that the weight rolls down the fingers as far as practical before they are curled closed. Maximally flex the wrist at the same time. In human movement terminology, these actions are finger and wrist flexion.

2. **Reverse Wrist Curls (Figure 7–56)**
    Target musculature: Wrist extensors
    Description: Grasp a dumbbell in the hand you wish to exercise first. Place the forearm and wrist, palm down, on the thigh of the same side as the wrist to be exercised. The hand and part of the wrist should extend beyond the knee. Drop the hand with the weight in it over the knee as far as practical before curling it back up to its most wrist-extended position. In human movement terminology, reverse curling of the wrist is *wrist extension.*

See Figures 7-57 and 7-58 for identification of the muscles you will use while weight/strength training.

REFERENCES

1. Pedersen, Nick, 1979. An electromyographic-electrogoniometric comparison: Free weight, Universal apparatus, Nautilus apparatus using selected muscles of the upper and lower extremities. Doctoral dissertation, Brigham Young University, Provo, Utah.

Figure 7–57
Anterior view of human
skeletal muscle

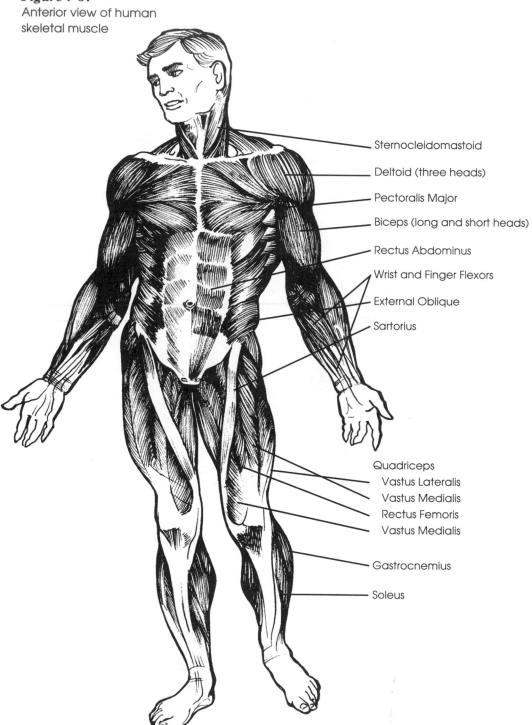

Sternocleidomastoid

Deltoid (three heads)

Pectoralis Major

Biceps (long and short heads)

Rectus Abdominus

Wrist and Finger Flexors

External Oblique

Sartorius

Quadriceps
  Vastus Lateralis
  Vastus Medialis
  Rectus Femoris
  Vastus Medialis

Gastrocnemius

Soleus

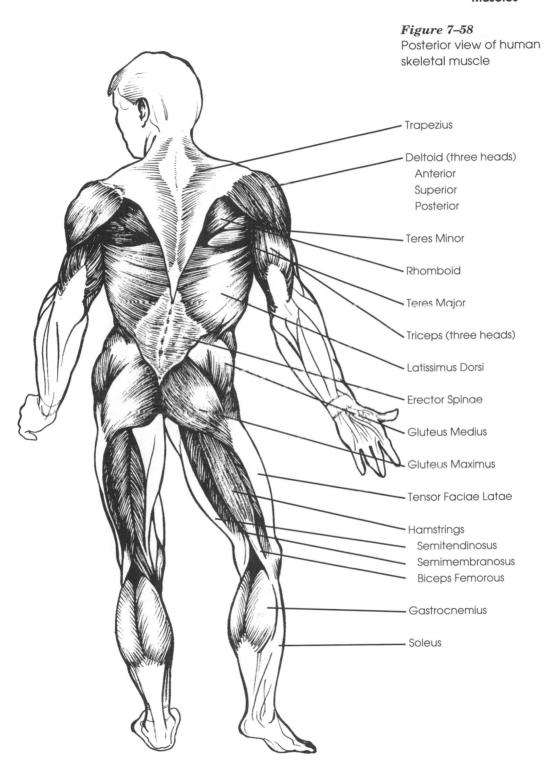

Figure 7–58
Posterior view of human
skeletal muscle

Trapezius

Deltoid (three heads)
  Anterior
  Superior
  Posterior

Teres Minor

Rhomboid

Teres Major

Triceps (three heads)

Latissimus Dorsi

Erector Spinae

Gluteus Medius

Gluteus Maximus

Tensor Faciae Latae

Hamstrings
  Semitendinosus
  Semimembranosus
  Biceps Femorous

Gastrocnemius

Soleus

CHAPTER EIGHT

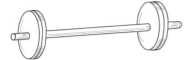

Evaluation

EVALUATION—A PERSPECTIVE

People who do not periodically evaluate themselves and the activities they engage in are likely to progress only marginally in life. One might suggest that the activities in which a person participates are the essence of that person. There is substance to that argument, but it is more true, in my opinion, that our real selves are more than our activities. Most of us have motivations, desires, drives, and awareness beyond the activities we are caught up in each day. Most frequently we are striving to become better at something, perhaps a number of things. Therefore, we need to take stock of how we are progressing.

Evaluation can become an unbearable burden if people have such high expectations of themselves that they must be the best at everything they try. Each of us should become very competent at some things in this life. Performing well in our occupations and within our families are two activities worthy of our very best. We will probably choose other activities (hobbies) to master, but an undeniable fact of life is that we do not have time to do everything the very best that it could possibly be done. Surely, when we engage in an activity, we should do the best we can with the time we have, but that does not imply we must reach expert status in everything. Therefore, when you evaluate yourself, be reasonable. Expect mastery at the highest levels in only those activities that you think are worthy of the time and effort for such achievement. Of course, it is also good to get a feel for our productivity. Are we getting the most out of our time? Or are we just frittering away time without the intensity that would produce the results we hope for?

Evaluation of your progress in weight training should be tempered with all the above considerations. If you happen to be interested in competitive weightlifting, evaluating your comparative ability is relatively simple. The records of those who have gone before you give ample evidence of great, good, and even poor performances. The performance of those who compete in advanced level bodybuilding, though not as easily judged as weightlifting, is also rather clear cut. But evaluating the results of time and effort spent in weight training for strength fitness presents some unique problems.

Most individuals who take up weight training would like to see and feel some increase in muscle tone, perhaps an improvement in body shape, and some increased strength and muscular endurance.

Have you ever seen a measure of muscle tone, or what I call *muscle fitness*? Some preliminary studies are being conducted that evaluate muscle density with ultrasound, but nothing has been done to relate density to muscular fitness (tone). Small changes in physique measurements usually require a great deal of time and effort, and getting before–after measurements demands that the exact same position on the body be measured with exactly the same tape pressure both times. These conditions are difficult to meet. Most instructors feel good about measurements for information purposes, but are reluctant to use them for evaluation.

As for strength and muscular endurance, admittedly measuring these characteristics and using the measurements as a basis for grading can be criticized. Students in a weight training class start at different levels; some are very capable and others are rank beginners. The potential gain in strength and muscular endurance varies from person to person. However, testing a combination of strength and muscular endurance offers the instructor the best means of evaluating the *practical* (physical achievement) progress of students in a weight training class.

Strength and muscular endurance can be evaluated isometrically, concentrically, and eccentrically, and machines or free weights can be used as the resistance. Of all the body characteristics, body weight correlates most closely with strength. Arrhenius tested the right and left leg flexion and extension strength of 302 athletes on the Cybex Orthotron. These strength measures were then correlated with body weight. The resulting correlation cooeficients for all athletes combined were .675 (left flexion), .689 (right flexion), .690 (left extension) and .711 (right extension) (1). These correlations do not suggest a perfect interrelationship between strength and body weight, but they are indicative of a reasonably strong association. Therefore, I use body weight as a basis for determining a person's relative strength.

There are two systems with which I have experimented. One is based on doing a specified number of repetitions (set), usually 10, with a certain percentage of body weight; the other is based on doing a set to failure using a certain percentage of body weight. The key in each of these cases is the percentage of body weight lifted. It has been my experience that students appreciate tests they think are fair. They generally like to know where they stand (as long as it isn't too low), and they enjoy the excitement of a performance test.

The percentage of body weight used for the repetition sets below have been developed over a number of years with information collected from hundreds of classes. The list of exercises for which data have been developed is not exhaustive. Some exercises are difficult to test (e.g., shrugs and toe presses), and reason suggests that beginning students not be required to do 10 repetition maximum sets of others (e.g., cleans).

My purpose in providing the following information is simply to offer help to those who may be wrestling with how to evaluate themselves or others.

TESTS REQUIRING A SPECIFIC NUMBER OF REPETITIONS— RESISTANCE LEVELS BASED ON BODY WEIGHT PERCENTAGES

Weight Training Score Sheet

Exercises requiring a *ten repetition set* are scored on the basis of *two points per repetition*. (Weight lifted should be as close to the exact percentage as possible—within 5–7 1/2 pounds). Dropping below the required resistance (weight) level results in a penalty as follows:

Minus 5 pound	=	1.5 points per repetition
Minus 10 pound	=	1.0 points per repetition
Minus 15 pound	=	0.5 points per repetition
Minus more than 15 pound	=	0 points

Students must use a weight with which they can do at least 5 repetitions.

Exercises that require more than 10 repetitions in a set are scored as follows:

Leg extensions	=	1 point per repetition
Bent leg sit-ups	=	.33 points per repetition
Back hyperextensions	=	0.5 points per repetition

For these exercises the required weight cannot be lowered.

Exercise	Req. for "A" reps M	F	Exact wt. for ea % bdy wt.	Actual wt. lifted	Reps.	Points	Verifying Initials

Phase I Test Exercises and Requirements

Exercise	Req. for "A" reps M	F	Exact wt. for ea % bdy wt.	Actual wt. lifted	Reps.	Points	Verifying Initials
Leg extensions	10	60%	45%				
Leg curls	10	47%	38%				
Bench presses	10	90%	52%				
Lat pulldowns	10	82%	62%				
Pullovers (Bent Arm)	10	64%	42%				
Shoulder presses (BB)	10	60%	40%				
Curls (BB)	10	60%	41%				
Tricep presses	10	42%	28%				
Back hyperextensions	50	Body wt. 2 min.					
Bent knee situps	100	Body wt. 2.5 min.					

Phase II Test Exercises and Requirements

Exercise	Req. for "A" reps M	F	Exact wt. for ea % bdy wt.	Actual wt. lifted	Reps.	Points	Verifying Initials
Leg presses	10	215%	190%				
Bench presses	10	93%	56%				
Cable rowing (Seated)	10	89%	70%				
Lat raises (Standing)	10	21%	15%				
Incline curls (DB)	10	24%	14%				
Tricep pressdowns	10	50%	35%				
Lunges	10	63%	53%				
Good morning exercises	10	63%	55%				
Crunch situps	80	Body wt. 2 min.					

Exercise	Req. for "A" reps M	F	Exact wt. for ea % bdy wt.	Actual wt. lifted	Reps.	Points	Verifying Initials

Phase III Test Exercises and Requirements

Exercise	Req. for "A" reps	M	F	Exact wt. for ea % bdy wt.	Actual wt. lifted	Reps.	Points	Verifying Initials
Leg presses	8	220%	200%					
Leg curls	8	48%	40%					
Incline presses (BB)	8	82%	63%					
Seated behind neck presses	8	60%	37%					
Curls (FCB on preacher bn.)	8	42%	23%					
Tricep pressdowns	8	60%	41%					
Bench presses (Nar. Grip)	8	65%	43%					
Crunch situps	95	Body wt. 2.5 min.						

Note that for each exercise there is only one requirement: percentage of body weight. This is the requirement for maximum credit, or an A. Any person relatively new to weight training (two to six months of exercise) who can complete all the exercises in the above tests, using the percentages listed, within a 50-minute time period, can consider him- or herself to have a high level of muscular strength and fitness.

For each of the tests, a student accrues a number of points. The maximum point value for Phase I is 228, for Phase II, 181, and for Phase III, 156. Instructors (or others) *can* gauge relative ability by simply calculating various percentages of the maximum points possible. A, B , C, or other grades *can* be given for various point totals.

Other criteria must also be met for the above evaluations to be valid. The two most important of these are:

1. All exercises must be done using strict form.
2. Each set must be done essentially all at once. Some struggle should be expected for the last repetition or two, but those taking the tests should do each set at a consistent cadence. For example, a set should

be one set of 8, 10, or 30 repetitions, not one set of 3 followed by seven sets of 1, or one set of 5, a set of 2, then three sets of 1 or the like. The difference between one set of 10 and one set of 3 followed by seven sets of 1 is, of course, *the rest time between repetitions.*

It is important for students in a weight training class be encouraged to do their very best. They should experience the difficulty of trying to complete a tough set. However, when taking one of the tests they need to give it their best only within certain reasonable guidelines. The reasonable guidelines are strict form and a consistent, rhythmic cadence. Not following the guidelines invalidates the test. Additionally, each of the tests above should be completed within one fifty-minute time period. Phase I can reasonably be given to beginners after a four-week, three-times-per-week workout regimen. Phase II can be given after about eight weeks, and Phase III after a twelve-week, three-workouts-per-week routine.

SET TO FAILURE TEST

Another method of testing a student's strength and muscular endurance is having him or her do a set to momentary muscular failure with a weight that is predetermined percent of body weight. The number of repetitions completed determines the level of achievement.

The following are the tests requiring sets to momentary muscuar failure.

Phase I (reasonable after a 5- to 6-week, 3-times-per-week workout regimen)

Exercise	Resistance Level		Excellent	Good	Fair	Poor
	Male	Female				
Leg extension	70%	60%	20 +	15–19	10–14	9 or less
Leg curls	46%	34%	20 +	15–19	10–14	9 or less
Bench presses	82%	46%	20 +	15–19	10–14	9 or less
Lat Pulldowns	83%	61%	20	15–19	10–14	9 or less
Pullovers (Bent arm)	55%	37%	20+	15–19	10–14	9 or less
Shoulder presses	53%	38%	20+	15–19	10–14	9 or less
Curls (Barbell)	50%	31%	20+	15–19	10–14	9 or less
Tricep presses (DB or FCB)	39%	23%	20+	15–19	10–14	9 or less

Phase II (reasonable after a 6- to 8-week, 3-times-per-week routine)

Exercise	Resistance Level					
	Male	Female	Excellent	Good	Fair	Poor
Leg press	1.95	1.70	20+	15–19	10–14	9 or less
Bench presses	85%	50%	20+	15–19	10–14	9 or less
Seated cable rowing	82%	62%	20+	15–19	10–14	9 or less
Lat raises (Standing/DB)	17%*	10%	20+	15–19	10–14	9 or less
Incline Curls (DB)	17%*	13%	20+	15–19	10–14	9 or less
Tricep pressdown	45%	31%	20+	15–19	10–14	9 or less
Lunges	57%	47%	20+	15–19	10–14	9 or less
Good morning exercises	55%	46%	20+	15–19	10–14	9 or less
Situps Body wt. (Bent knee)	100 +	85–99	61–84	60 or less		

* The percentage of body weight to be in *each* hand

Phase III (Reasonable after an 8- to 10-week, 3-times-per-week regimen)

Exercise	Resistance Level					
	Male	Female	Excellent	Good	Fair	Poor
Leg presses	200%	180%	20+	15–19	10–14	9 or less
Leg curls	48%	35%	20+	15–19	10–14	9 or less
Incline presses (Barbell)	62%	43%	20+	15–19	10–14	9 or less
Bent over rowing	45%	31%	20+	15–19	10–14	9 or less
Seated behind neck presses	40%	25%	20+	15–19	10–14	9 or less
Preacher bn curls	26%	15%	20+	15–19	10–14	9 or less
Tricep pressdowns	47%	33%	20+	15–19	10–14	9 or less
Bench presses (nar grip)	57%	38%	20+	15–19	10–14	9 or less
Crunch situps	Body wt.	95+	80–94	65–79	50–64	

When students who have taken both tests (the Specific Number of Reps Test above and the Set to Failure Test) are asked which they prefer, the response has been about 50-50. Some students cannot do even 1 repetition of some of the exercises on the Specified Repetition Test. Thus one advantage of the Set to Failure Test Format is that everyone can usually do at least some repetitions with the test weight. The pain produced when doing a set to failure is the major drawback of that test.

Once again I want to remind you that the resistance levels and repetition requirements in this chapter should be used only as a guide. The tests should be given a thorough trial on the equipment available in your weight rooms before considering them as a basis for grading. I believe that the standards for exercises requiring free weights, when done using correct technique, are quite good. The exercises requiring machines may, because of differences in machines, have little validity for you.

Evaluation of one's ability can result in happiness and self-satisfaction, or feelings of inadequacy and failure. It is generally thought that we must experience the latter to appreciate the former. Assuming this thesis is correct, it is my wish that on only one occasion will negative feelings be your lot, and that all other times of evaluation bring you joy and contentment with your significant achievements.

REFERENCES

1. Arrhenius, A. 1978. Knee flexion and extension: The establishment and comparison of strength norms among college athletes. Masters thesis, Brigham Young University, Provo, Utah.

Index